THE RIGHT TEST

A Physician's Guide to Laboratory Medicine

CARL E. SPEICHER, M.D.
Professor and Director, Clinical Laboratories,
Ohio State University, Columbus, Ohio

1989
W. B. SAUNDERS COMPANY
Harcourt Brace Jovanovich, Inc.

Philadelphia, London, Toronto, Montreal, Sydney, Tokyo

'IDERS COMPANY

:ace Jovanovich, Inc.

Center
ice Square West
iia, PA 19106

Library of Congress Cataloging-in-Publication Data

Speicher, Carl E.
    The right test.

    Bibliography: p.
    Includes index.
    1. Diagnosis, Laboratory—Handbooks, manuals, etc.
I. Title.
RB38.2.S64   1989   616.07'5   89-10540
ISBN   0-7216-3065-0

Editor: John Dyson

THE RIGHT TEST: A Physician's Guide
to Laboratory Medicine   ISBN   0-7216-3065-0

Printed in the United States of America.

Last digit is the print number :   9   8   7   6   5   4   3   2   1

TO OUR PATIENTS

ACKNOWLEDGMENT

I am grateful to my colleagues and students at Ohio State University as well as to my associates across the country for their help in formulating the ideas expressed in this book. Special thanks are extended to Donald A. Senhauser, M.D., for sharing his view of laboratory medicine with me and providing the environment to do my work; to Thomas D. Stevenson, M.D., for his invaluable medical expertise and judgment; to Chris Anderson for her meticulous attention to each and every aspect of committing these concepts to paper; and to John Dyson for his unhesitating, enthusiastic, and friendly support on behalf of the W. B. Saunders Company.

CARL E. SPEICHER, M.D.

PREFACE

Like others who have struggled to learn the rules of English grammar and punctuation, I have turned for help to the "little book" of Strunk and White called *The Elements of Style*.[1] In contrast to the formidable volumes that were presented to us during our school years, this "little book" is more friendly and gently guides us with succinct recommendations and explanations on how to write and punctuate. Strunk and White's approach is to take a position on a particular issue and indicate that position, often in the form of an imperative statement, recognizing fully that experienced writers can take liberties with the recommendations to create a more interesting writing style.

It occurred to me that Strunk and White's format might be useful for presenting a concise approach to medical decision making using laboratory tests, that is, how to choose the right tests, how to evaluate the tests, how to tell the difference between true-positive and -negative and false-positive and -negative results, and how to monitor the patient's condition.

I decided to use the format of Strunk and White for describing an approach to using laboratory tests in the context of medical problem solving. Although there are no standards, I have taken a position for using laboratory tests in each decision-making situation. It is not my intention to say that the positions in this book are the only way to make particular medical decisions but simply that they are one good way. Certainly there are others. Like the experienced writer, the experienced physician, in the context of clinical judgment, can take liberties with the recommendations to do what is best for the individual patient.

The reader is encouraged to peruse the Introduction, which immediately follows. By doing this, the organization of the text will become apparent, and maximal benefit will be attained.

REFERENCE

1. Strunk W, White EB: The Elements of Style, 3rd ed. New York, Macmillan Publishing Co, 1979.

CONTENTS

INTRODUCTION

The problem-solving, medical decision-making approach used in this book relies on theoretical concepts that were developed in a previous work, *Choosing Effective Laboratory Tests.*[10] Readers interested in these concepts, such as statistical and representation techniques useful in medical decision making, are referred to this prior source. These techniques can help to clarify and quantify medical decisions.

Since there are already over 1000 available laboratory tests and the number of tests is constantly increasing, trying to learn about tests one by one can be a frustrating, time-consuming task. On the other hand, the number of clinical problems that rely on laboratory tests for their solution is much smaller and should be easier to learn. Learning about a relatively small number of common clinical problems and the component medical decisions should enable us to effectively deal with most clinical situations where laboratory tests are important. Clearly, the point of departure in choosing laboratory tests is the clinical history and physical examination. In the context of differential diagnosis, laboratory tests should be chosen like a rifle, not a shotgun, to confirm or exclude a given diagnosis.[4] In this book, common clinical problems were selected that rely significantly on laboratory tests for their solution.[3,7]

The physician's task of managing a particular patient's problem is composed of a series of discrete medical decisions. Some decisions rely heavily on laboratory test results for their solutions; some decisions use test results as ancillary information to clinical, radiographic, or electrocardiographic data; and other decisions do not depend on laboratory data at all. The effective use of laboratory data can be better understood in the context of discrete medical decisions. For example, in the setting of the hospital coronary-care unit, serial measurements of serum creatine kinase–MB (CK-MB) have high sensitivity and specificity for diagnosing acute myocardial infarction. In contrast, the sensitivity and specificity of a single measurement of CK-MB for determining the same diagnosis in the setting of the emergency department are much lower because, constrained by time, there is usually the opportunity to obtain only a single measurement of CK-MB.[2] Not only a medical problem-solving, but also a medical decision-making, approach is used in this book.

In practice, medical decision making by physicians using laboratory tests is often not very scientific, and there are significant opportunities for improvement. Physicians learn their test-ordering behavior according to protocols or routines that are the product of accumulated anecdotal experience, are sanctioned by general use, and appear to have the weight of authority. Guidance on diagnostic testing in medical textbooks often consists of little more than listings of tests that may be abnormal in a given disease. Good, scientifically based protocols for test ordering in common medical decision-making situations are needed.[12] Potential source material for such protocols includes literature data, expert opinion, consensus conferences, recommendations of learned societies, metaanalysis in which results from a number of literature reports are combined to yield a single conclusion, and clinical studies. In a recent study, it was possible to decrease inappropriate serum triiodothyronine (T_3) testing by 38% and thyrotropin (thyroid-stimulating hormone or TSH) testing by 61% simply by implementing a decision-based test request form for hyperthyroidism and hypothyroidism in place of a menu of individual thyroid tests. This maneuver accomplished the reduction by eliminating inappropriate testing, such as excessive ordering of the TSH test and the T_3 test. Moreover, physicians were assured of obtaining the correct tests for the diagnosis they had in mind.[13]

Development of problem-solving, medical decision-making test request and report systems is a particularly promising method to enhance appropriate laboratory testing. Not only does it help to ensure that appropriate tests are requested and unnecessary tests are eliminated, but also it offers the opportunity to efficiently introduce new and better tests, eliminate the tests that are replaced, and ensure that the full information content of the test results is clearly communicated to the requesting physician.

Sometimes, in spite of one's best efforts, it is difficult to obtain a consensus of opinion concerning the testing strategy that is appropriate for a given medical decision-making situation; that is, the issue is controversial. For example, since the therapy of asymptomatic hyperparathyroidism is controversial, is it worthwhile to screen asymptomatic individuals for hypercalcemia?

PROBLEM ORGANIZATION

In this book, each clinical problem is discussed in terms of individual medical decisions: when to choose certain tests and which tests to choose, how to evaluate the tests, what to do if test results are positive, what to do if test results are negative, and how to use tests to monitor the patient if the diagnosis is confirmed. The format is to state the decision recommendation in bold type, followed by a justification of the recommendation in regular type.

The Introduction

In the introduction, the problem is defined, and its importance is discussed. Information on the prevalence and incidence is provided, if available. The discussion includes some pathophysiologic concepts, as well as a consideration of the main causes or origins of the problem. Then, some notion of the relative importance of laboratory tests compared to clinical, radiographic, and other data is given. Key clinical findings may be summarized.

Which Tests to Choose

In this section, information is provided concerning appropriate tests to request in a given screening or diagnostic situation. In addition, there is a brief explanation of the reasons for obtaining these tests. Sometimes, tests that should not be obtained are also mentioned. Unfortunately, in practice, the use of a new test does not usually tend to replace the other tests for which it provides an alternative. Rather, the new test is often "piggybacked" onto the old tests.[6]

If patient preparation or specimen collection and handling issues are important, instructions are provided on how to perform these tasks properly. For example, accurate measurement of the plasma partial thromboplastin time depends on filling the citrated collection tube completely with blood, thoroughly mixing it, and promptly delivering it to the laboratory.

How to Evaluate the Tests

Physicians should learn more about laboratory tests. The clinical laboratory is not simply a "black box" where one requests tests and always receives equivalent results. There are pitfalls related to specimen collection and handling, methodologies, and the skills of the individuals performing the tests. All laboratory tests are not created equal, and test differences can affect results, which in turn can affect medical decisions.[9] Greater knowledge about laboratory tests not only will enable physicians to use tests more effectively, but also will help them to better understand the nuances of office laboratory testing and home (self) testing. In some situations, it may occasionally be helpful for physicians to actually know how to perform some tests themselves: (1) preparation and examination of a Gram-stained smear of the sputum for pneumonia and of the urine for urinary tract infection, (2) performance of a macroscopic (dipstick) urinalysis and microscopic examination of the urinary sediment for urinary tract disorders, and (3) preparation and examination of a Wright-stained peripheral blood smear for anemia. For certain medical decisions, it is imperative to know not only which test or tests to request but also which method or methods to use and how the methods should be standardized and controlled. For example, one cannot use the National Institutes of Health (NIH) recommendations for desirable, borderline-high, or high levels for serum cholesterol unless one uses a method for measuring cholesterol that is equivalent to the NIH method.[11] It is also important to know the diagnostic utility of tests, that is, how effective they are in confirming or excluding a diagnosis.[6] Recently, a five-phase process was suggested to assess the clinical utility for a diagnostic marker test.[5]

Physicians should use the reference ranges of the laboratory that performs their tests. Common reference ranges are provided inside the front and back covers of this book, and special reference ranges are included in the test evaluation section of each problem. Reference ranges and other laboratory values are given in conventional units followed by international units in parentheses. Appropriate reference ranges should address important variables (analytic; biologic, genetic, and ethnic; environmental; and life-style).

Information on clinical decision levels is also included in this section. The term "decision level" refers to a threshold value above which or below which a particular management action is recommended. The use of decision levels recognizes the importance and additional information content in knowing not only whether a test result is high or low, but also how high or how low. For example, the reference range (normal range) for serum calcium is 8.4 to 10.2 mg/dl (2.10 to 2.55 mmol/L). The decision level above which hypercalcemic coma can occur is 13.5 mg/dl (3.37 mmol/L), and the decision level below which tetany can occur is 7.0 mg/dl (1.75 mmol/L). It would be inappropriate to assign the cause of a patient's coma to hypercalcemia if the level was 11.5 mg/dl (2.87 mmol/L), since, even though 11.5 mg/dl is above the upper limit of the reference range for serum calcium, it is below the decision level for hypercalcemic coma.[VII]

How to Interpret Positive and Negative Test Results

In this section, information is provided on the sensitivity and specificity of test results in regard to the disease or disorder under consideration. Take thyroid function tests for the diagnosis of hyperthyroidism or hypothyroidism, for example. A serum thyroxine (T_4), a triiodothyronine resin uptake (T_3RU), and a calculated free thyroxine index (FT_4I) are only about 95% sensitive for hyperthyroidism, and if the T_4 and FT_4I are normal in the presence of clinical findings suggestive of hyperthyroidism, a serum triiodothyronine (T_3) or the new highly sensitive immunoradiometric assay for thyrotropin, the S-TSH, is indicated to confirm the diagnosis. On the other hand, a serum T_4 or FT_4I is even less sensitive to detect hypothyroidism, and if the T_4 and FT_4I are normal in the face of clinical features of hypothyroidism, a serum TSH or S-TSH is indicated to confirm the diagnosis.

If a test result does not make sense or is indeterminate, a useful tactic is to repeat it. For example, when testing for human immunodeficiency virus (HIV) infection, if the enzyme-linked immunoassay (ELISA) is positive and the Western blot analysis is indeterminate, repeat the Western blot test monthly.

How to Monitor the Patient's Disorder

Finally, if a diagnosis is confirmed and the patient is treated, this section gives information on which tests are useful to monitor the patient's condition and how often these tests should be ordered. For example, in patients with acute hepatitis B who are e antigen positive, it is appropriate to test for anti–hepatitis B e antibody monthly, since development of the antibody will indicate when the patient is less infectious to others.

Additional Abnormal Test Results

Sometimes, test results are available that are not really necessary for the diagnostic strategy but have been ordered as part of a profile or for some other reason. It is important to know whether or not these test results can occur in the condition under consideration and whether or not one has to hypothesize another disease process to explain them. If available, information on the pathophysiologic derangements responsible for these abnormal test results is also included here.

Instead of an alphabetical listing of tests and their reference range values, the abnormal test results are organized conceptually according to the way the results are usually grouped and considered. This same organization is used for common reference ranges located inside the front and back covers of this book.

ADDITIONAL CONSIDERATIONS

There are data in the medical literature that support the approach used in this book, that is, a series of recommendations followed by an explanation of the underlying reasons. It seems that individuals have difficulty with rote memorization of recommendations, unless the reasons for the rules are understood. Further, physicians will not use rules for medical decision making unless they have confidence that the rules are correct. This confidence comes from an understanding of the underlying reasons.[1,8]

Material for this book comes from three sources: the author's experience, general references at the end of the book, and particular references at the end of each problem. The particular references were chosen mainly to highlight important information that has surfaced between the publication of the general references and the present time.

Finally, it is hoped that a more scientific approach to medical decision making using laboratory tests will help assure the quality of patient care. This quality assurance through appropriate laboratory testing is not only good for patients but also is economical. Moreover, physicians' anxiety about medicolegal risk should be lessened, because, to the extent possible, the recommendations in this book are based on the best information currently available.

REFERENCES

1. Elstein AS, Shulman LS, Sprafka SA: Medical Problem Solving. An Analysis of Clinical Reasoning. Cambridge, Mass, Harvard University Press, 1978, p 199.
2. Lee TH, Goldman L: Serum enzyme assays in the diagnosis of myocardial infarction. Recommendations based on a quantitative analysis. In Sox HC (ed): Common Diagnostic Tests. Use and Interpretation. Philadelphia, American College of Physicians, 1987, p 19.
3. Marsland DW, Wood M, Mayo F: Content of family practice. J Fam Pract 3:37, 1976.
4. Moser R: No more "battered" patients: Blue Cross urges curb on hospital tests. Time, February 19, 1979, p 80.
5. Nierenberg AA, Feinstein AR: How to evaluate a diagnostic marker test. Lessons from the rise and fall of dexamethasone suppression test. JAMA 259:1699, 1988.
6. Robin ED: Of hydras, lemmings, and diagnostic tests. Arch Intern Med 147:1704, 1987.
7. Rosenblatt RA, Cherkin DC, Schneeweiss R, et al: The structure and content of family practice. Current status and future trends. J Fam Pract 15:681, 1982.

8. Schwartz S, Griffin T: Medical Thinking. The Psychology of Medical Judgment and Decision Making. New York, Springer-Verlag, 1986, p 169.
9. Speicher CE: All laboratory tests are not created equal. Arch Pathol Lab Med 109:709, 1985.
10. Speicher CE, Smith JW: Choosing Effective Laboratory Tests. Philadelphia, WB Saunders Co, 1983.
11. The Expert Panel: Report of the national cholesterol education program expert panel on detection, evaluation, and treatment of high blood cholesterol in adults. Arch Intern Med 148:36, 1988.
12. Wong ET, Lincoln TL: Ready! Fire! . . . Aim! An inquiry into laboratory test ordering. JAMA 250:2510, 1983.
13. Wong ET, McCarron MM, Shaw ST: Ordering of tests in a teaching hospital. Can it be improved? JAMA 249:3076, 1983.

THE RIGHT TEST

A Physician's Guide to Laboratory Medicine

CHAPTER 1

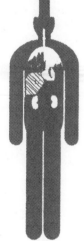

WELLNESS SCREENING AND CASE FINDING

In over 0.5 million family practice patient visits, the periodic health examination was the most common reason (8.4%) why individuals visited their physician,[6] and laboratory tests play a key role in this kind of patient evaluation. It is important to distinguish patients who are asymptomatic from patients who are symptomatic or have a disease. Asymptomatic patients are basically healthy, and the testing of these individuals has been referred to as wellness screening. Case finding is the detection of disease in patients seen for unrelated symptoms or diseases.[3] Therefore the screening of ambulatory patients can be either wellness screening or case finding, depending on whether or not the patient is symptomatic. On the other hand, hospital preadmission or admission screening is, by definition, case finding, since the patients are symptomatic. The underlying strategy for screening by laboratory tests relies on the difference between wellness screening and case finding. In wellness screening, individuals at risk should be evaluated using reliable tests for diseases that represent a significant health hazard and for which effective therapy is available: for example, serum cholesterol as a risk factor for coronary heart disease and a Pap test for cancer of the uterine cervix. In wellness screening, it is appropriate to restrict certain kinds of testing to individuals of a particular age or sex or with specified risk factors. For example, occult fecal blood testing for colorectal carcinoma is appropriate for individuals after 50 years of age, and testing for sexually transmitted diseases is recommended in sexually active patients with multiple partners.[7] In case finding, patients may be tested for disorders that are unrelated to their present illness. When the cause of the patient's illness is unclear, the screening should be more thorough and vigorous, because laboratory testing may discover information that is undetected by clinical findings.[4]

Some benefits of screening that are difficult to document include (1) baseline studies with which to compare future test results (changes or trends often being more important than a single value), (2) reassurance that the patient is free of disease,[17] and (3) the fact that the performance of groups of tests or profiles often costs less than several individual tests (in large laboratories, groups of tests or profiles are often cheaper than a small number of tests individually performed because groups of tests or profiles are batched and automatically performed).

Wellness screening and case finding are often done by groups of tests called profiles. Historically, profiles were groups of tests determined quite simply on the basis of which tests a given laboratory instrument could perform or which tests were more commonly ordered, for example, the classic 12-test biochemical profile. Laboratories should optimize their profiles, so that the test content is determined on the basis of medical decision-making needs rather than instrument capabilities or the frequency of tests. It is the content of the profile—not the concept of the profile—that has been problematic.[3,4]

1. In wellness screening, request a complete blood count (CBC), urinalysis, biochemical tests, and other analyses when the individual examined belongs to a clinical class that is at risk for significant conditions that may be manifested by abnormalities in these tests. Otherwise, do not routinely request tests (and profiles) without a good reason.

The main idea in wellness screening is to test patients who are at risk for diseases for which effective therapy is available. Mindless, routine testing creates the opportunity for false-positive test results and fruitless follow-up testing with little real gain. Baseline information against which to compare future test results, data for the physician that make other tests unnecessary, and reassurance that the patient is free of disease are legitimate reasons for requesting screening tests.[3,4]

Examples of individuals who have a high prevalence of anemia and who may benefit from a CBC include infants in the first year of life; institutionalized, elderly persons; pregnant women; and recent immigrants from third world countries.[12] A mild iron deficiency anemia may provide the first clue to colorectal carcinoma in an otherwise healthy older individual. In recognition of the fact that a CBC is often performed on an automated instrument that usually gives values for hemoglobin, hematocrit, red cell indices, and leukocytes —and sometimes platelets and an electronic differential as well—one simply orders a CBC. On the other hand, if you are only interested in detecting anemia and a discrete hemoglobin or hematocrit measurement is available, you may wish to request a hemoglobin or hematocrit. Similarly, you may wish to obtain only a manual leukocyte count and differential.

Consider measuring serum cholesterol in adults 20 years of age and over because of the high prevalence of hypercholesterolemia as a risk factor for coronary heart disease.[2] Although screening for gestational diabetes is beneficial, routine screening for diabetes in the nonpregnant adult may not be very productive. Screening for diabetes might be reasonable for particular patients, for example, obese persons who would be spurred to lose weight by a demonstration of glucose intolerance.[13] Although some experts believe that screening serum calcium or uric acid determinations are valuable, others argue that there is no advantage in treating asymptomatic hyperparathyroidism or hyperuricemia and therefore that screening for these analytes should be omitted. The American College of Physicians endorses screening asymptomatic persons using serum glucose, cholesterol, and creatinine (with or without urea nitrogen).[1,4,5]

Examples of individuals who have a high prevalence of urinary tract disorders and who may benefit from a urinalysis include pregnant women, older men with prostatic hypertrophy and obstruction, and anyone known to have a history of recurrent urinary tract disease. Because a urine dipstick test (including nitrite and leukocyte esterase) is such an effective and economical way to detect urinary tract diseases that cause serious morbidity, it may be appropriate to incorporate it into the routine physical examination to detect covert pyuria, hematuria, and proteinuria.[14]

Consider requesting thyroid function tests to detect a cause for hypercholesterolemia[2] or to detect thyroid dysfunction in older individuals in whom the prevalence of thyroid disorders is increased and symptoms are unreliable.[4,15] Since the prevalence of sexually transmitted diseases is increasing, consider testing for *Chlamydia* and gonorrhea in sexually active patients with multiple partners.[8-10] Urine screening for drug abuse is an area of increasing interest,[11] and screening for alcohol abuse and human immunodeficiency virus (HIV) infection is also important. Consider testing adult women for cervical cancer using the Pap test and older individuals for colorectal carcinoma using the occult fecal blood test.[4]

2. In case finding, request tests that are appropriate for the clinical situation.

In case finding, appropriate testing depends on the good judgment of the attending physician. Testing may range from a few tests to a wide variety of routine and special laboratory studies. If an otherwise healthy patient is seen with a minor injury or for an elective minor surgical procedure, little testing may be necessary.[16] On the other hand, a diabetic patient with ketoacidosis requires a large number of tests to diagnose and manage the immediate problem, as well as to look for coexisting conditions and complications, such as urinary tract infection. As in wellness screening, baseline information, reassurance of normality, and data that make other tests unnecessary are appropriate reasons for requesting tests.[3,4]

3. Interpret test results in the context of the complete general health examination.

Clinical laboratory test results are valuable, but they are only one part of the assessment of patients and are best used in the context of other examinations such as: (1) the general history and physical examination, (2) blood pressure, (3) weight, (4) hearing and vision, (5) oral examination, (6) breast examination, (7) electrocardiogram, (8) mammography, (9) sigmoidoscopy, and (10) radiographs.

Abnormal results should be followed up with additional testing. Sometimes, an abnormal test result will be found that does not make sense in the context of the clinical findings, and one wonders whether it is correct. This situation constitutes the unexplained test result, which should be approached as out lined in the next discussion.

REFERENCES

1. Campion EW, Glynn RJ, DeLabry LO: Asymptomatic hyperuricemia: Risks and consequences in the normative aging study. Am J Med 82:421, 1987.
2. The Expert Panel: Report of the national cholesterol education program expert panel on detection, evaluation, and treatment of high blood cholesterol in adults. Arch Intern Med 148:36, 1988.
3. Gambino R: The American College of Physicians and Blue Cross/Blue Shield guidelines. Lab Report for Physicians 10:44, 1988.
4. Gambino R: Biochemical profiles: Applications in ambulatory screening and preadmission testing of adults. In Glenn GC (ed): Blue Cross/Blue Shield Guidelines based on Common Diagnostic Tests. Use and Interpretation. Skokie, IL, College of American Pathologists, 1988, p 20.

5. General Internal Medicine Subspeciality Committee: Medical Knowledge Self Assessment Program VIII. General Internal Medicine. Philadelphia, American College of Physicians, 1988, p 18.
6. Marsland DW, Wood M, Mayo F: Content of family practice. J Fam Pract 3:37, 1976.
7. Mulley AG: Screening tests for the healthy patient. Med Clin North Am 71:625, 1987.
8. Phillips RS, Aronson MD, Taylor WC, et al: Should tests for *Chlamydia trachomatis* cervical infection be done during routine gynecologic visits? An analysis of the costs of alternative strategies. Ann Intern Med 107:188, 1987.
9. Phillips RS, Hanff PA, Wertheimer A, et al: Gonorrhea in women seen for routine gynecologic care: Criteria for testing. Am J Med 85:177, 1988.
10. Sadof MD, Woods ER, Emans J: Dipstick leukocyte esterase activity in first-catch urine specimens. A useful screening test for detecting sexually transmitted disease in the adolescent male. JAMA 258:1932, 1987.
11. Saxon AJ, Calsyn DA, Haver VM, et al: Clinical evaluation and use of urine screening for drug abuse. West J Med 149:296, 1988.
12. Shapiro MF, Greenfield S: The complete blood count and leukocyte differential count. An approach to their rational application. In Sox HC (ed): Common Diagnostic Tests. Use and Interpretation. Philadelphia, American College of Physicians, 1987, p 133.
13. Singer DE, Samet JH, Coley CM, et al: Screening for diabetes mellitus. Ann Intern Med 109:639, 1988.
14. Sodeman TM: Urinalysis and urine culture in women with dysuria. In Glenn GC (ed): Blue Cross/Blue Shield Guidelines based on Common Diagnostic Tests. Use and Interpretation. Skokie, IL, College of American Pathologists, 1988, p 15.
15. Tibaldi JM, Barzel US, Albin J, et al: Thyrotoxicosis in the very old. Am J Med 81:619, 1986.
16. Turnbull JM, Buck C: The value of preoperative screening investigations in otherwise healthy individuals. Arch Intern Med 147:1101, 1987.
17. Werner M, Altshuler CH: Utility of multiphasic biochemical screening and systematic laboratory investigations. Clin Chem 25:509, 1979.

THE UNEXPLAINED TEST RESULT

Unexplained abnormal test results may occur in the context of wellness screening or case finding. These unexplained test results may not indicate disease but may simply result from incorrect patient preparation, poor specimen collection and handling, laboratory error, use of inappropriate reference ranges, or statistical outliers. Sometimes, they are due to drugs or life-style effects. On the other hand, they may be truly indicative of disease. The strategy for investigating an unexplained abnormal test result is to first determine whether the result is simply an error or whether it is truly abnormal and possibly indicative of disease. Follow-up studies should be done only if the result suggests disease.[2]

1. If a slightly abnormal test result does not fit with the patient's clinical and other laboratory findings, consider that it may represent a statistical outlier that may be ignored.

Minor test result "abnormalities" are common during wellness screening and case finding. These results are statistical outliers that may often be ignored if they lie just outside the normal range (>2 but <3 standard deviations) and the patient has no other clinical, radiographic, or laboratory findings. The probability of occurrence for these statistical outliers increases with the number of different tests performed as follows[1]:

NUMBER OF TESTS	PERCENTAGE OF PERSONS WITH ABNORMAL RESULTS*
1	5
6	24
12	43

*Using the mean ±2 standard deviations for the normal range.

2.   If, however, an abnormal test result might be more than a minor statistical outlier and could have real clinical significance, for example, elevated serum calcium, verify the result rather than ignoring it. Pay attention to significantly abnormal test results.

It is important to distinguish test results that are markedly abnormal from those that are minimally abnormal (possible statistical outliers); that is, pay attention to the strength of the signal. Human immunodeficiency virus (HIV) testing is a good example to illustrate this important point. A weak HIV antibody signal (titer) in a low-risk group is almost always a false-positive result, since the probability of disease is only 0.0007%. On the other hand, a strong HIV antibody signal among military recruits is predictive of disease 96.9% of the time.[3,5]

A general approach to determine whether an unexplained test result abnormality indicates disease is as follows[VI*]:

1.   Repeat the measurement (only repeat tests that are abnormal, i.e., if a 12-test biochemical profile reveals an abnormal serum calcium, only repeat the serum calcium measurement, not the entire 12-test biochemical profile).
   a.   Prepare the patient properly.
   b.   Obtain a proper sample.
   c.   Ensure appropriate specimen handling.
   d.   Use the best laboratory method available (e.g., for serum calcium, use the atomic absorption method, if available).

2.   Use the proper reference range for the age and sex of the patient.

3.   If the abnormal test result has been verified, consider a drug effect or a life-style effect, and if this does not explain the abnormality, consider the significance of the abnormal test result in the context of the individual's clinical and other laboratory findings.

A common example of an unexplained test result is an elevated serum alkaline phosphatase (ALP).[6,7] Occasionally, the elevation can be explained by a specimen collection and handling problem or a laboratory error, or sometimes the patient will be found to be a growing child or a pregnant woman, which will explain the elevated result. Sometimes, the elevation will be found to be due to a drug effect that may occur with agents such as chlorpromazine or methyltestosterone. The elevation can be caused by ALP forming a macroenzyme

*Roman numeral reference numbers refer to the general references at the end of the book.

complex with immunoglobulin, and the elevation can persist for years and has no clinical significance. This phenomenon can also occur with amylase, creatine kinase, lactate dehydrogenase, alanine aminotransferase, and glucose-6-phosphatase dehydrogenase.[4]

Life-style effects can be due to such things as exercise, alcohol intake, and smoking. For example, vigorous exercise in an unconditioned person can elevate serum creatine kinase; excessive alcohol intake can cause anemia, elevated lipids, and numerous other test abnormalities; and smoking can elevate serum carcinoembryonic antigen (CEA). Marathon runners, after the completion of a race, may have hematuria and a positive test for fecal occult blood. If enough blood is lost, anemia can occur.

Only if an unexplained test result, such as a high serum ALP, cannot be accounted for by factors such as those discussed above should one consider a differential diagnosis and follow-up studies. Unrecognized disease may be the cause for an unexplained abnormality, such as Paget's disease for an unexpected elevation of ALP.[2,6,7]

The significance of an unexplained test result may be clarified by considering it in the context of the patient's clinical and other laboratory findings. For example, an unexplained elevation of serum ALP in an elderly man with a history of prostatic carcinoma takes on a special significance because the patient is at risk for metastatic bone disease, which may be manifested by an elevated serum ALP. Similarly, if an unexplained elevation of ALP occurs in a middle-aged, overweight woman who also has a mildly elevated serum bilirubin, the possibility of cholelithiasis comes to mind and additional studies are appropriate.

REFERENCES

1. Barnett RN: Clinical Laboratory Statistics, ed 2. Boston, Little, Brown & Co, 1979, p 171.
2. Belsley R, Speicher CE, Winkelman J: Lab results that don't fit the picture. Patient Care 21:40, 1987.
3. Gambino R: The American College of Physicians and the Blue Cross/Blue Shield guidelines. Lab Report for Physicians 10:44, 1988.
4. Litin SC, O'Brien JF, Pruett S, et al: Macroenzyme as a cause of unexplained elevation of aspartate aminotransferase. Mayo Clinic Proc 62:681, 1987.
5. Schwartz JS, Dans PE, Kinosian BP: Human immunodeficiency virus test evaluation, performance, and use. Proposals to make good tests better. JAMA 259:2574, 1988.
6. Speicher CE: Unexplained elevation of alkaline phosphatase. Clinical Chemistry No CC-81-2. Chicago, American Society of Clinical Pathologists, 1981.
7. Wolf PL: Clinical significance of an increased or decreased serum alkaline phosphatase level. Arch Pathol Lab Med 102:497, 1978.

PREGNANCY TESTING

Modern pregnancy tests do not simply test for pregnancy: they test for either the beta subunit of human chorionic gonadotropin (hCG) using an immunoassay or for the hCG molecule itself using a monoclonal antibody. These newer tests eliminate false-positive test results caused by elevated thyrotropin (thyroid-stimulating hormone [TSH]), follicle-stimulating hormone (FSH), and luteinizing hormone (LH). In practice, the distinction between hCG and LH is most important because the normal midcycle surge in LH that triggers ovulation can be mistakenly identified as hCG in nonspecific pregnancy tests. These newer tests are more specific than older tests for hCG, which use polyclonal antibodies, and pregnancy can be detected at an earlier date with fewer false-positive results. Human chorionic gonadotropin is secreted by the trophoblastic tissue of the placenta of the developing pregnancy into the pregnant woman's serum and is then excreted in the urine. It becomes detectable within 24 hours after implantation of the fertilized ovum and peaks at about 10 weeks after the last menstrual period. Human chorionic gonadotropin increases regardless of whether the fetus and trophoblastic tissue are developing in the uterus or elsewhere, such as in the fallopian tube (ectopic pregnancy). Trophoblastic and other tumors can also secrete hCG and cause false-positive pregnancy tests.[2]

1. Perform a urine or serum pregnancy test to screen for or to confirm the diagnosis of pregnancy. Perform a serum pregnancy test if the earliest possible detection of pregnancy is important, if an ectopic pregnancy is suspected, or if there is any question about the validity of a previous urine pregnancy test. Serial quantitative serum hCG determinations are useful to diagnose ectopic pregnancy.

Modern pregnancy tests for serum or urinary hCG are very sensitive and specific. Several points should be kept in mind: (1) use serum or a concentrated first-morning urinary specimen collected in a clean, dry container; (2) carefully label the specimen; and (3) promptly deliver the specimen to the laboratory.

If you are performing the test yourself or in your office, (1) choose a kit that uses a monoclonal antibody to hCG; (2) make certain the test kit has been stored properly and is not outdated; (3) choose a kit that incorporates controls; (4) meticulously follow the directions; and (5) perform the test promptly.

2. Evaluate the tests.

URINE PREGNANCY TEST

Newer methods, which use monoclonal antibody to hCG, are preferred. Urine pregnancy tests are qualitative—the results are either positive or negative. The most sensitive methods give positive results at the time of the first missed menstrual period, and most methods give positive results within 2 to 3 weeks after the first missed period. Blood, protein, or detergents in the urine are potential causes of interference with the test.

SERUM PREGNANCY TEST

Methods using antibody to beta-hCG or monoclonal antibody to hCG are best. Serum pregnancy tests may be either qualitative or quantitative. Serum hCG becomes detectable within 24 hours after implantation (5 mIU/ml), increases progressively, and reaches levels of 100 to 500 mIU/ml at 30 days, 50,000 to 140,000 mIU/ml at 10 weeks, and 10,000 to 50,000 mIU/ml after 16 weeks. Higher than expected levels may be found in multiple pregnancies, polyhydramnios, eclampsia, and erythroblastosis fetalis. Ectopic pregnancy can be suspected if serum hCG fails to rise to levels seen in a normal pregnancy and if the rate of rise is less than that of a normal pregnancy. The absence of a uterine gestational sac with levels above 6500 mIU/ml is associated with an ectopic pregnancy in 87% of the cases; however, only 40% of patients with a suspected ectopic pregnancy have an hCG titer above 6500 mIU/ml. In the latter situation, serial hCG determinations to determine an abnormal rate of increase are useful for diagnosing ectopic pregnancy. A normal intrauterine pregnancy should have at least a 66% increase of serum hCG over a 48-hour observation period. A lower rate of increase would indicate an abnormal pregnancy in 85% of cases, whereas a higher rate might indicate a multiple pregnancy.[3,5-7]

Serum hCG can be elevated in the following conditions[1]:

• Normal pregnancy
• Ectopic pregnancy
• Abortion
• Gestational trophoblastic tumors: hydatiform mole and choriocarcinoma
• Testicular tumors, germinal cell origin: choriocarcinoma, embryonal carcinoma with syncytiotrophoblastic giant cells, and seminoma with syncytiotrophoblastic giant cells
• Other tumors: some gastric carcinomas, some pancreatic carcinomas, and other tumors

3. Remember that either false-positive or false-negative results can occur.

Many companies manufacture tests for hCG. These tests are marketed for use in clinical laboratories, physicians' offices, or patients' homes (self tests). They vary in price and ease of use, but the bottom line is the same—most of them are good tests based on the same good technology. These modern pregnancy tests use antibodies that have sensitivities for hCG in serum or urine as low as 20 to 50 mIU/ml or lower. The lower the level of hCG that can be detected, the earlier the pregnancy can be diagnosed, that is, before, at, or shortly after the first missed menstrual period.

Modern pregnancy tests have a number of pitfalls that may cause false-positive or false-negative results, and it is important to be aware of these pitfalls so that they can be avoided. Correct labeling of the patient's specimen is the first important step. Women with abdominal pain have been operated for ectopic pregnancy only to find that they were not pregnant and that their positive pregnancy test result was due to a mix-up with a pregnant woman's sample. Second, a concentrated urine sample is best, because the concentration of urinary hCG approximates the concentration of serum hCG only if the urine is concentrated. Thus urinary pregnancy tests are best performed on first-morning urinary specimens, which are usually concentrated. Random urinary specimens are often quite dilute, with a concentration of hCG that is significantly less than serum. These dilute urinary specimens may result in false-negative results in early pregnancy. Clinical laboratories are turning to serum pregnancy tests to avoid this problem. One way to avoid false-negative results from dilute urinary specimens is to measure the specific gravity of the urinary specimen and not do the pregnancy test if the urinary specimen is dilute. The urinary specimen should be collected in a clean, dry container, since detergents or other contaminants may interfere with the test. Moreover, the urinary specimen should be tested promptly, and if this is not possible, the specimen should be covered and refrigerated. Another pitfall is related to the integrity of the test reagents. Most test kits will say when they are outdated, as well as conditions under which the test kit should be stored. If the test kit is outdated or if there is any question that the kit has been improperly stored, do not use it. Even with a good urinary specimen and sound test kit reagents, mistakes may still occur. Some mistakes occur because the test is improperly performed. The directions must be carefully read and meticulously followed. It is also better to choose a test kit that incorporates controls. Positive and negative controls establish that the test system is working properly. Other mistakes occur when a woman performs a pregnancy test in her own home (home test or self test). Her vested interest in the result may cause subjective bias, and mistakes may occur (9.5% of layperson results were discrepant with one test kit and 12.5% with another).[4]

Finally, remember that even if you consider all these things, false-positive and false-negative results may occasionally occur. There is no perfect pregnancy test.

4. In pregnant women, the following abnormal laboratory test results may occur:

HEMATOLOGY

- Decreased hemoglobin and hematocrit related to increased plasma volume that can be aggravated by iron deficiency anemia.
- Leukocytosis during late pregnancy and labor. Myelocytes can be found in the peripheral blood in pregnancy.
- Thrombocytopenia.

CHEMISTRY

- Decreased PCO_2 from respiratory alkalosis caused by an increasing enlargement of the uterus and a stimulating effect on respiration by pregnancy hormones.
- Hyperglycemia from glucose intolerance caused by ovarian and placental hormones.
- Decreased urea nitrogen because of expanded intravascular space and increased glomerular filtration rate: a decreased urea nitrogen/creatinine ratio (below 10:1).
- Decreased creatinine. A creatinine of 1.2 mg/dl (106.1 μmol/L) or greater in pregnancy represents an elevated level.
- Decreased uric acid.

- Hyponatremia caused by expanded intravascular space.
- Increased chloride caused by decreased bicarbonate secondary to respiratory alkalosis, which is especially prominent during labor.
- Decreased total CO_2 caused by respiratory alkalosis.
- Hypocalcemia related to insufficient ingestion of calcium, phosphorus, and vitamin D.
- Hypophosphatemia, slight, with no significant implications.

- Increased creatine kinase (CK) during last few weeks and remains elevated during parturition, becoming normal 5 days postpartum.
- Decreased CK during eighth to twentieth week with minimal level at twelfth week.
- Decreased aspartate aminotransferase (AST or SGOT) caused by decreased pyridoxine during pregnancy.
- Increased lactate dehydrogenase (LD).
- Increased alkaline phosphatase from the placenta. First appears in second trimester, increases in third trimester, and disappears 4 weeks postpartum.

- Hypoalbuminemia caused by expanded intravascular space.
- Hypercholesterolemia, probably related to increased hepatic synthesis.

REFERENCES

1. Bakerman S: ABC's of Interpretive Laboratory Data, 2nd ed. Greenville, NC, Interpretive Laboratory Data Inc, 1984, p 239.
2. Bluestein D: Monoclonal antibody tests. AFP 38:197, 1988.
3. Daya S: Human chorionic gonadotropin increase in early pregnancy. AM J Obstet Gynecol 156:286, 1987.
4. Hicks JM, Iosefsohn MI: Reliability of home pregnancy test kits in the hands of laypersons. N Engl J Med 320:320, 1989.
5. Kadar N, Caldwell BV, Romero R: A method for screening for ectopic pregnancy and its indications. Obstet Gynecol 58:162, 1981.
6. Norman RJ, Buck RH, Rom L, et al: Blood or urine measurement of human chorionic gonadotropin for detection of ectopic pregnancy? Obstet Gynecol 71:315, 1988.
7. Romero R, Kadar N, Copel JA: The value of serial human chorionic gonadotropin testing as a diagnostic tool in ectopic pregnancy. Am J Obstet Gynecol 155:392, 1986.

THE PAP TEST AND CANCER OF THE UTERINE CERVIX

About 15,000 women develop carcinoma of the uterine cervix in the United States each year, and approximately 7000 die from the disease. Screening for carcinoma of the cervix has decreased the incidence of cervical cancer and reduced the mortality by 50%. About 2.5 cases of carcinoma of the cervix are detected for every 10,000 vaginal smears examined. The strategy that follows reflects recommendations of the American Cancer Society, the American College of Obstetricians and Gynecologists, the American Medical Association, and the National Cancer Institute. Major factors affecting the effectiveness of the strategy are the technique of the physician who takes the Papanicolaou

(Pap) smear and the competency of the laboratory that analyzes it. Recently, human papillomavirus (HPV) has been associated with cervical cancer. Testing for this virus may prove to be a more sensitive tactic to detect patients with the disease than Pap tests.[5,6]

1.   Perform initial cervical cytologic screening using good technique in all women 18 years of age and older and in those women who have been sexually active regardless of age.

Poor technique is a significant cause of false-negative Pap tests. Some of the more common causes of poor smears are (1) a thick smear from an abundance of red blood cells or inflammatory cells; (2) poor fixation, often caused by air drying the smear before fixation; (3) a scarcity of cells, caused by wiping the cervix before obtaining the smear; and (4) an absence of endocervical cells that results from failure to obtain an endocervical sample.[1]

2.   Consider testing for HPV in cervical smear and biopsy specimens as tests become available. On the basis of currently available information, women with cervical abnormalities should receive evaluation, treatment, and follow-up using current Pap test and biopsy technology for these abnormalities independent of the presence or absence of HPV.

HPV is a DNA virus that has been implicated as a cause of cervical cancer, and koilocytotic change is a cytologic finding that can signal the presence of viral infection. Although it remains to be proven, five specific types of HPV (types 16, 18, 31, 33, 35) have been found in cervical cells of 90% to 95% of women with cervical cancer. Type 18 is especially prevalent in fast-growing cancers. Types 6 and 11, although not linked to cancers, are often found in abnormal-looking cervical cells. HPV is the fastest-rising sexually transmitted disease in the United States. The possibility of false-negative Pap tests is a strong stimulus for developing HPV tests. The reported sensitivity of the Pap test for cervical cancer and precursor lesions is as low as 70% and may never be much above 95% even under the most ideal conditions. A commercial HPV test kit for types 6, 11, 16, 18, 31, 33, and 35 is available.* An HPV test or an HPV test and a Pap test may eventually prove to have a higher sensitivity for cancerous or potentially malignant cervical lesions than a Pap test alone, so that fewer false-negative results would occur and women who should be closely monitored can be identified.[2-4,7]

3.   Obtain cervical cytologic reports that evaluate the Pap test in terms of diagnostic implications rather than arcane numerical systems.

The American Society of Cytology and the International Academy of Cytology recommend a format such as the one that follows[1]:

DIAGNOSTIC TERMINOLOGY IN CERVICAL CYTOLOGY

Unsatisfactory (cite reason and recommendation)

No abnormal cells

---

*Vira Pap® (Life Technologies, Inc., Gaithersburg, MD)

Mild squamous atypia
> Metaplasia
> Inflammation (with organism if identified)
> Regeneration and repair
> Radiation effect
> Viral effect
> Other (specify)

Cytologic findings consistent with dysplasia
> Mild
> Moderate
> Severe (carcinoma in situ)

Cytologic findings consistent with invasive squamous cell carcinoma

Abnormal cells not specifically categorized

4. Evaluate every significantly abnormal result. A single negative report on a repeat smear does not eliminate the need for a thorough diagnostic evaluation.

The diagnostic evaluation should include visual inspection, colposcopically directed biopsy, endocervical curettage, and when indicated, cervical conization. Although Schiller's test may be of benefit in directing attention to abnormal areas of the cervix and particularly the vagina, the inaccuracy of using this technique alone has been reported. Random or four-quadrant biopsies appear to be even less reliable. In Schiller's test the cervical and vaginal epithelium are painted with a solution of iodine. Glycogen-rich normal epithelium takes on a mahogany color. Dysplastic epithelium and carcinoma in situ appear pale or unstained.[1,5]

5. If the cervical cytologic report is normal, repeat cervical cytologic screening annually. Following therapy for preinvasive and invasive malignancy, repeat screening every 3 months for 2 years and then every 6 months.

The American Cancer Society and the American College of Obstetricians and Gynecologists have recently recommended that if three successive annual Pap smears are negative, starting when the individual reaches age 18 years or becomes sexually active, then, at the discretion of the physician, the woman may have the tests less frequently. These guidelines have also been adopted by the National Cancer Institute and the American Medical Association.[6]

6. In patients with carcinoma of the cervix, the following abnormal results may occur:

- Increased lactate dehydrogenase (LD).
- Increased alkaline phosphatase (ALP). As a group, cancer of the ovary, endometrium, cervix, and breast exhibits the highest frequency of the Regan isoenzyme.
- Increased carcinoembryonic antigen (CEA).

REFERENCES

1. American College of Obstetricians and Gynecologists: Cervical cytology: Evaluation and management of abnormalities. Washington, DC, ACOG Technical Bulletin 81, October 1984.
2. Bonfigli TA, Stoler MH: Human papillomavirus and cancer of the uterine cervix. Hum Pathol 19:62, 1988.
3. Gambino R, Krieger P: False-negative fractions in cytology screening. Lab Report for Physicians 10:61, 1988.
4. Gay JD, Donaldson LD, Goellner JR: False-negative results in cervical cytologic studies. Acta Cytologica 29:1043, 1985.
5. Koss LG: The Papanicolaou test for cervical cancer detection. A triumph and a tragedy. JAMA 261:737, 1989.
6. Medical groups reach compromise on frequency of giving pap tests. *New York Times,* January 7, 1988, p 10.
7. Medical News and Perspectives: DNA probes for papillomavirus strains readied for cervical cancer screening. JAMA 260:2777, 1988

ELEVATED SERUM CHOLESTEROL AND CORONARY HEART DISEASE

Coronary heart disease (CHD) causes more than 550,000 deaths in the United States each year, and up to 50% of the population may have elevated serum cholesterol levels that place them at increased risk for the disease. Up to 25% may be at high risk. The assumption is that each 1% reduction in serum cholesterol will reduce the CHD rate by 2% with possible reductions up to 50% in individuals with other risk factors. The recommendations that follow are essentially those of the National Cholesterol Education Program Expert Panel.[9] They have been endorsed by the American Heart Association.[1] These recommendations should be placed in the context of other sound health promotion measures such as smoking prevention and cessation, blood pressure control, reduction of alcohol and drug abuse, correction of gross obesity, and appropriate exercise. Not everyone agrees with these recommendations. For example, it has been suggested that the less stringent recommendations of the Consensus Conference of 1985, using the 75th and 90th percentiles for serum cholesterol for moderate- and high-risk levels, were sufficient.[6,16] In the final analysis, clinical judgment, based on assessment of all risk factors present in an individual patient, patient compliance, and the risk-to-benefit ratio, remains the hallmark of clinical practice and therapeutics.[16,17]

1.   Measure serum cholesterol in every adult 20 years of age and over — whether the patient is fasting or nonfasting — at the time of the first visit. Measure serum cholesterol in children who have a strong family history of elevated cholesterol or CHD. Do not screen for elevated cholesterol in patients who are acutely ill or pregnant, and do not screen patients with serum apolipoprotein studies or lipoprotein electrophoresis.

Serum or heparinized plasma may be used. Blood should be drawn in the absence of venous stasis, since stasis can increase cholesterol concentration (e.g., after a tourniquet is applied for 5 minutes, cholesterol can increase 5% to 10%). Good technique is important when collecting blood by skin puncture (e.g., excessive milking of the skin can significantly lower the cholesterol concentration because of dilution with tissue fluids). Serum cholesterol is quite stable at room temperature, but if delays in testing are anticipated, the specimen should be refrigerated.

The serum cholesterol level is not significantly elevated after a meal; therefore the blood specimen may be drawn any time the patient is seen. Since cholesterol levels may be affected by an acute medical or surgical illness, they should not be measured in patients who are ill. Patients who are evaluated should be ambulatory, in their usual state of health, on their normal diet, and not pregnant.

The guidelines for detection and management of hypercholesterolemia for children are not as clear as for adults. The American Academy of Pediatrics suggests that children (2 years and older) at high risk should be identified primarily by carefully obtained family histories that include parents, grandparents, and all first-degree relatives. A family history of hypercholesterolemia or premature CHD should alert the physician to obtain at least two serum cholesterol determinations and a lipid analysis. Others believe that all children should be screened. A recent University of Michigan study found that 25% of children have cholesterol levels above 180 mg/dl (4.66 mmol/L). In rural schoolchildren, 40% were above that level. Some researchers suggest that levels above 180 mg/dl in children indicate increased risk of high cholesterol levels in adulthood.[12]

The serum cholesterol in the first 24 hours after myocardial infarction reflects preinfarction levels. The optimal time to determine the cholesterol levels in these patients is immediately after the patient is first seen.[13]

Serum apolipoprotein A-1 and the ratio of apolipoprotein A-1 to apolipoprotein B may be better markers for CHD than serum lipids. Currently, measurements of serum apolipoproteins require better standardization, reference ranges, and relevant information about treatment programs that can modify apolipoprotein levels. Until these improvements can be accomplished, serum lipids are more appropriate for screening programs.[15,17]

Lipoprotein electrophoresis is not recommended as a screening test. It can be useful in the diagnosis of certain lipid disorders, such as abetalipoproteinemia, Tangier disease, broad-beta disease, lipoprotein lipase deficiency, and lipoprotein x in cholestasis.

2. Evaluate the tests.

Recommendations for Classification of Adults Serum Total Cholesterol [9]

<200 mg/dl (5.17 mmol/L): desirable blood cholesterol
200-239 mg/dl (5.17-6.18 mmol/L): borderline-high blood cholesterol
≥240mg/dl (6.21 mmol/L): high blood cholesterol

To properly use these reference ranges, your laboratory's results must be accurate, that is, appropriately standardized with the reference method of the Centers for Disease Control (CDC) or the National Bureau of Standards (NBS).* Ask your laboratory how its cholesterol method is standardized, and if you

---

*National Institute for Standards and Technology (NIST) as of September, 1988.

measure cholesterol in your office, ask the same question of the manufacturer of your office method.[3-5] If your laboratory results do not perfectly agree with the reference method, a correction factor can be used. The College of American Pathologists, through its surveys, can assist laboratories in standardizing their methods.* The national reference method for measuring cholesterol is the CDC method, which is traceable to the NBS method. The reproducibility or precision of the cholesterol method is also important. The Laboratory Standardization Panel on Blood Cholesterol Measurement of the National Cholesterol Education Program (NCEP) recommends that imprecision be reduced to a coefficient of variation (CV) of 5% or less at this time and to less than 3% by 1993 and that inaccuracy be reduced to below ±5% from the true value at this time and to below ±3% by 1993.[7]

Children with serum cholesterol levels between the 75th and 90th percentiles, 170 to 185 mg/dl (4.40 to 4.78 mmol/L), should have a lipid analysis and be counseled regarding their diet and other cardiovascular risk factors and then observed at 1-year intervals. Those with levels above the 90th percentile, 185 mg/dl (4.78 mmol/L), require special dietary instruction and close supervision with evaluation of other risk factors. A child with a serum cholesterol level above the 95th percentile, 200 mg/dl (5.17 mmol/L), on two occasions is in a special category and should be checked for hereditary hypercholesterolemia. Such a child should be given the same vigorous dietary and pharmacologic treatment given the adult. Dietary management of children with elevated serum cholesterol levels should be part of total management that includes regular exercise programs, maintenance of ideal weight, and avoidance of excess salt and cigarette smoking. All family members should be screened.[2,6,12]

In public screening programs, all individuals with a serum cholesterol level of 200 mg/dl (5.17 mmol/L) or greater should be referred to their physician for remeasurement and evaluation. Remember that all serum cholesterol levels should be confirmed by repeat measurements, with the average used to guide clinical decisions. Baseline lipid values are best determined by averaging two to three measurements, 1 to 8 weeks apart. If the initial serum cholesterol value is 200 mg/dl (5.17 mmol/L) or greater, the individual should return in 1 to 8 weeks for confirmation. If the confirmation value is within 30 mg/dl (0.78 mmol/L) of the first test, the average of the two results is used to guide subsequent decisions. If the second value differs from the first by over 30 mg/dl, a third test should be obtained in another 1 to 8 weeks and the three values averaged.

In patients with hyperlipidemia, the following additional abnormal laboratory test results may occur.

CHEMISTRY

- Hyperuricemia
- Artifactual hyponatremia (pseudohyponatremia) caused by lipemia (In artifactual hyponatremia the serum osmotic pressure is normal.)
- Hypercalcemia associated with an increase in the calcium bound to lipoproteins

---

*Write to College of American Pathologists, 5202 Old Orchard Rd, Skokie, Il 60077.

- Hypoalbuminemia with possible elevations of beta and gamma-globulin fractions

3. If the serum cholesterol level is below 200 mg/dl (5.17 mmol/L), remeasure within 5 years or with subsequent physical examination. In individuals with a cholesterol of 200 to 239 mg/dl (5.17 to 6.18 mmol/L), no CHD*, and not more than one additional risk factor, remeasure annually and prescribe a step-1 diet.† Provide dietary and risk factor education.

The serum cholesterol level can vary with age, diet, weight, physical activity, and medications, and it is prudent to remeasure the level periodically. Additional risk factors include:

- Male sex
- Family history of premature CHD (definite myocardial infarction or sudden death before 55 years of age in a parent or sibling)
- Cigarette smoking (currently smokes more than 10 cigarettes per day)
- Hypertension
- Low HDL-cholesterol concentration (<35 mg/dl [<0.91 mmol/L])‡
- Diabetes mellitus
- History of definite cerebrovascular or occlusive peripheral vascular disease
- Severe obesity (≥30% overweight)

4. If serum cholesterol is 240 mg/dl (6.21 mmol/L) or above or if it is 200 to 239 mg/dl (5.17 to 6.18 mmol/L) and the patient has CHD† or two or more additional risk factors, remeasure and order a serum lipid analysis, including total cholesterol, LDL-cholesterol, HDL-cholesterol, and triglycerides. The patient must fast at least 12 hours before blood is drawn for the repeat studies.

Recommendation for Classification of Adults[9]

Serum LDL-Cholesterol§
<130 mg/dl (3.36 mmol/L): desirable LDL-cholesterol
130–159 mg/dl (3.36–4.11 mmol/L): borderline-high LDL-cholesterol
≥160 mg/dl (4.14 mmol/L): high LDL-cholesterol

---

*CHD equals history of myocardial infarction or definite myocardial ischemia, such as angina pectoris.

†A step-1 diet is essentially the same as the American Heart Association diet for the public.[1]

‡Consider measuring the HDL-cholesterol concentration in individuals who are likely to have a low level. There are a number of causes for a reduced serum HDL-cholesterol level, some of which are reversible: heavy cigarette smoking, obesity, lack of exercise, hypertriglyceridemia, anabolic steroids, progestational agents, antihypertensive agents, and genetic factors, e.g., primary hypoalpha-lipoproteinemia. White men, but not necessarily black men, have lower HDL-cholesterol levels than women. If HDL-cholesterol is low, try to elevate it by managing the above variables. Drug therapy is not indicated.[1,11]

§Two measurements of LDL-cholesterol after an overnight fast are made 1 to 8 weeks apart, and the average is used for clinical decisions unless the two values differ by more than 30 mg/dl (0.78 mmol/L). In which case a third test is carried out, and the average of all three is used. If the triglycerides are below 400 mg/dl, calculate LDL-cholesterol as follows (all quantities are in milligrams per deciliter: LDL-cholesterol = Total cholesterol − HDL-cholesterol − (0.16 × Triglycerides).[8]

HDL-Cholesterol

≥35 mg/dl (≥0.91 mmol/L): desirable HDL-cholesterol

Triglycerides

<250 mg/dl (2.82 mmol/L): desirable triglycerides
250–500 mg/dl (2.82–5.65 mmol/L): borderline hypertriglyceridemia
≥500 mg/dl (5.65 mmol/L): hypertriglyceridemia

The usual serum cholesterol measurement estimates total cholesterol, which is mainly composed of LDL-cholesterol and HDL-cholesterol. LDL-cholesterol carries cholesterol to the atherosclerotic plaques in the arteries, and HDL-cholesterol removes it. It has been shown that lowering LDL-cholesterol and raising HDL-cholesterol not only can prevent but also potentially reverse plaque formation. Serum triglycerides do not constitute a significant risk factor for heart disease but are an important part of the total lipid profile. There is little evidence that triglyceride levels below 250 mg/dl (2.82 mmol/L) in the presence of a normal cholesterol predict an increased risk of any disease. However, very high triglycerides (1000 mg/dl [11.30 mmol/L] or above) are associated with pancreatitis. Hypertriglyceridemia is frequently associated with obesity, uncontrolled diabetes mellitus, liver disease, alcohol ingestion, and uremia as well as with the use of estrogen-containing contraceptives, steroids, isoretinoin, and antihypertensive agents.

One of the commonest problems with obtaining valid serum lipid studies is failure of the patient to observe the 12-hour fast.

5.   If serum LDL-cholesterol is below 130 mg/dl (3.36 mmol/L), remeasure within 5 years. If serum LDL-cholesterol is 130 to 159 mg/dl (3.36 to 4.11 mmol/L) and there are less than two additional risk factors and no CHD, remeasure annually and prescribe a step-1 diet. Provide dietary and risk factor education.

Low serum cholesterol may be a sign of good health, proper diet, and appropriate exercise. On the other hand, it may signal disease, since the following disorders can be associated with low cholesterol: severe liver damage, hyperthyroidism, malnutrition, chronic anemia, and malignancy. Drugs, such as cortisone and ACTH therapy, are an additional cause of low cholesterol.

6.   If serum LDL-cholesterol is 160 mg/dl (4.14 mmol/L) or above or if it is 130 to 159 mg/dl (3.36 to 4.11 mmol/L) and the patient has CHD or two or more additional risk factors, then evaluate the patient for secondary hypercholesterolemia caused by diabetes mellitus, hypothyroidism, cholestasis, the nephrotic syndrome, dysproteinemia, and drugs. If a responsible disease or drug is the cause, treat the disease or remove the drug.

Exclude diabetes mellitus with a fasting blood glucose, hypothyroidism with a serum thyroid-stimulating hormone (TSH), cholestasis with liver function tests, the nephrotic syndrome with a urinary protein determination, and dysproteinemia with a serum protein electrophoresis. Drugs, such as oral contraceptives, progestins, and anabolic steroids, can elevate serum cholesterol.

Antihypertensive medications have the following effects: thiazides and loop diuretics increase triglycerides, total cholesterol, and LDL-cholesterol with no change or a lowering of HDL-cholesterol; beta-adrenergic antagonists increase triglyceride and decrease HDL-cholesterol levels (a reciprocal rise in LDL-cholesterol causes total cholesterol to remain the same); and alpha-adrenergic antagonists decrease triglyceride, increase HDL-cholesterol, and possibly decrease LDL-cholesterol.[14] Check any drugs that the patient is taking for a possible hypercholesterolemic effect. When one of the causes of secondary high cholesterol is present, the usual approach is to treat the disease or discontinue the drug (if possible) and then to reevaluate the LDL-cholesterol level.

7. If a cause for secondary hypercholesterolemia is not present, consider familial dyslipidemias, including familial hypercholesterolemia (FH).

The triad of hypercholesterolemia, xanthomas, and a familial incidence is typical of FH. The xanthomas are caused by deposits of cholesterol-laden macrophages. Cholesterol deposits can also occur in the eyelids and corneas, but unlike xanthomas over tendons, deposits in the eyelids and corneas are not typical of FH. FH is due to a genetically determined deficiency of LDL-cholesterol cell receptors. The receptors clear LDL-cholesterol from the plasma and thus lower serum cholesterol. Heterozygotes have half the normal number of LDL-cholesterol receptors, and their serum cholesterol is approximately twice normal. Homozygotes have even fewer LDL receptors, and their serum cholesterol is about four times normal. By age 60 years, 80% of heterozygotes have had a myocardial infarction. Homozygotes have their infarcts at an earlier age. About 1 in every 500 persons has heterozygous FH. Homozygous FH is much less common. Most individuals with hypercholesterolemia have neither FH nor another disease as the cause of their hypercholesterolemia; that is, their hypercholesterolemia is primary and idiopathic. It may soon be possible to diagnose FH by measuring LDL-cholesterol cell receptors on circulating lymphocytes.

Other familial dyslipidemias should be considered: polygenic (severe primary) hypercholesterolemia, familial combined hyperlipidemia (FCHL), familial dysbetalipoproteinemia (type 3 hyperlipoproteinemia), familial hypertriglyceridemia (FHTG), familial type 5 hyperlipoproteinemia, and familial type 1 hyperlipoproteinemia. Because an accurate diagnosis may be required for correct treatment of the patient, physicians may desire to refer patients suspected of having familial dyslipidemia to a lipid specialist.[1]

8. After considering secondary hypercholesterolemia and familial dyslipidemia, if LDL-cholesterol is 160 mg/dl (4.14 mmol/L) or above (cholesterol of 240 mg/dl [6.21 mmol/L] or above) or if LDL-cholesterol is 130 to 159 mg/dl (3.36 to 4.11 mmol/L) (cholesterol of 200 to 239 mg/dl [5.17 to 6.18 mmol/L]) and the patient has CHD or two or more additional risk factors, prescribe a step-1 diet. Remeasure cholesterol in 4 to 6 weeks and at 3 months.

For individuals with less than two additional risk factors and no CHD, the goal is to reduce serum cholesterol to below 240 mg/dl (6.21 mmol/L) and LDL-cholesterol to below 160 mg/dl (4.14 mmol/L). For individuals with CHD or two or more additional risk factors the target for serum cholesterol is below

200 mg/dl (5.17 mmol/L) and for LDL-cholesterol below 130 mg/dl (3.36 mmol/L). Individuals with additional risk factors need to achieve lower values since, for example, the risk of a level of 200 mg/dl (5.17 mmol/L) in a smoker is roughly equivalent to the risk of 275 mg/dl (7.11 mmol/L) in a nonsmoker.[10]

If goals are not achieved by 3 months, refer the individual to a registered dietitian and remeasure cholesterol in 4 to 6 weeks and at 3 months after retrial on a step-1 diet and then after trial on a step-2 diet. Continue dietary therapy under a registered dietitian for at least 6 months before considering drug treatment. Shorter periods can be considered for patients with severe elevations of LDL-cholesterol above 225 mg/dl (5.82 mmol/L) or those with established CHD. When a decision is made to use drugs, maximal dietary therapy should be continued.[1]

9. If the serum cholesterol goal is achieved, confirm that the LDL-cholesterol goal is achieved, and monitor serum cholesterol four times in the first year and two times per year thereafter. Reinforce dietary and behavior modification.

Reducing the patient's cholesterol level toward 200 mg/dl (5.17 mmol/L) will help prevent premature CHD, and reducing it toward lower levels will reduce the risk even further. Appropriate goals are the reduction of serum cholesterol to below 180 mg/dl (4.66 mmol/L) for subjects under 30 years of age, and to below 200 mg/dl (5.17 mmol/L) for subjects over 30 years of age.

10. If the serum cholesterol and LDL-cholesterol goals are not achieved following a minimum of 6 months of dietary therapy under a registered dietitian, review the medical history, continue dietary therapy, and commence drug treatment for patients with LDL-cholesterol of 190 mg/dl (4.92 mmol/L) or above or 160 to 189 mg/dl (4.14 to 4.89 mmol/L) and CHD or two or more additional risk factors.

Remeasure LDL-cholesterol in 4 to 6 weeks and at 3 months. If the LDL-cholesterol goal is achieved, monitor total cholesterol every 4 months and remeasure LDL-cholesterol annually. If the LDL-cholesterol goal is not achieved, use another drug or combination treatment or consult with or refer the patient to a lipid specialist if drug treatment is not successful. In women, a more conservative approach to drug therapy is appropriate, because the absolute risk of CHD is lower in women than in men.

11. After prescribing drug therapy, monitor the patient for possible adverse effects of cholesterol-lowering drugs.

For example, for patients taking lovastatin, monitor liver function tests every 4 to 6 weeks during the first 15 months of therapy with lovastatin and periodically thereafter.

REFERENCES

1. American Heart Association: Physicians' Cholesterol Education Handbook. Recommendations for the Detection, Classification, and Treatment of High Blood Cholesterol. AHA National Center, Dallas, 1988.

2. Barness LA: Cholesterol and children. JAMA 256:2871, 1986.
3. Blank DW, Hoeg JM, Kroll MH, et al: The method of determination must be considered in interpreting blood cholesterol levels. JAMA 256:2867, 1986.
4. Boyd JC: Accuracy in cholesterol assays. Clin Chem 34:2194, 1988.
5. Burke JJ, Fischer PM: A clinician's guide to the office measurement of cholesterol. JAMA 259:3444, 1988.
6. Consensus Conference: Lowering blood cholesterol to prevent heart disease. JAMA 253:2080, 1985.
7. Current status of blood cholesterol measurement in clinical laboratories in the United States: A report from the laboratory standardization panel of the national cholesterol program. Clin Chem 34:193, 1988.
8. DeLong DM, DeLong ER, Wood PD, et al: A comparison of methods for the estimation of plasma low- and very low-density lipoprotein cholesterol: The Lipid Research Clinics' prevalence study. JAMA 256:2372, 1986.
9. The Expert Panel: Report of the national cholesterol education program expert panel on detection, evaluation, and treatment of high blood cholesterol in adults. Arch Intern Med 148:36, 1988.
10. Grundy SM: Cholesterol and coronary heart disease. A new era. JAMA 256:2849, 1986.
11. Grundy SM, Goodman DS, Rifkind BM, et al: The place of HDL in cholesterol management. A perspective from the National Cholesterol Education Program. Arch Intern Med 149:505, 1989.
12. High cholesterol found in children. *New York Times*, October 10, 1988, p 19.
13. Jackson R, Scragg R, Marshall R, et al: Changes in serum lipid concentrations during the first 24 hours after myocardial infarction. Br Med J 294:1588, 1987.
14. Lardinois CK, Neuman SL: The effects of antihypertensive agents on serum lipids and lipoproteins. Arch Intern Med 148:1280, 1988.
15. Naito HK, Galen RS: Apolipoproteins: Biochemistry, physiology, and pathophysiology. Clinical Chemistry No CC85-3. Chicago, American Society for Clinical Pathology, 1985.
16. Palumbo PJ: National cholesterol education program: Does the emperor have any clothes? Mayo Clin Proc 63:88, 1988.
17. Rifkind BM, Lippel K (eds): Cholesterol Screening. Clinics in Laboratory Medicine, Philadelphia, WB Saunders Co, 9(1): March, 1989.

OCCULT FECAL BLOOD TESTING AND COLORECTAL CARCINOMA

In the United States, colorectal carcinoma is the second leading cause of carcinoma, and the incidence of carcinoma of the large intestine was 140,000 in 1986. The prevalence of detectable cancer in a previously unscreened population is about 3 to 4 per 1000 persons above the age of 45 years, and this prevalence increases with age. Current thinking suggests that a high-fiber, low-fat diet will help prevent the disease. Using the following strategy for occult fecal blood testing to detect colorectal carcinoma about 2% to 6% of asymptomatic individuals over 50 years of age will have a positive test result. The false-positive rate is acceptably low, but the false-negative rate is significant: it is higher for colonic polyps than for cancer. Occult fecal blood testing has higher sensitivity for right-sided lesions than for cancer in the left side, perhaps because of greater blood loss from right-sided cancers. Failure to meticulously observe a protocol such as the one that follows will increase both false-positive and false-negative results. Patient compliance in returning the test cards is often poor. The evidence to date suggests that occult fecal blood testing will reduce morbidity and mortality from colorectal carcinoma. Because occult fecal blood testing has relatively low sensitivity, clinical clues, such as anemia, bleeding, changes in bowel movements, and pain, must not be neglected.*

1.   Perform annual fecal occult blood testing to screen for colorectal carcinoma using Hemoccult II® (SmithKline Diagnostics, Inc., Philadelphia) in all asymptomatic persons as early as 46 years of age and no later than 50 years of age. Patients with a family history or a personal history of colorectal neoplasia or ulcerative colitis and patients with positive clinical findings require more aggressive diagnostic studies.

Hemoccult II® is the test of choice, because it has been validated with other reference techniques—such as labeling erythrocytes with chromium 51 to detect blood loss—and has achieved widespread acceptance. Blood losses greater than 20 ml/day are necessary to achieve 80% to 90% sensitivity for a Hemoccult test.[5] It requires at least 60 ml, and more likely over 100 ml, to make the stool black.[11]

The Canadian Task Force on the Periodic Health Examination suggests annual stool occult blood testing for persons after 46 years of age. The American Cancer Society suggests it for persons after 50 years of age and annual digital rectal examination after 40 years of age.[2]

2.   To perform fecal occult blood testing, place the individual to be tested on a diet† 2 days before the first stool collection and continue this diet throughout the collection period. Instruct the individual concerning specimen collections.

The individual should be instructed as follows:

- Beginning on the third day of the diet, take two specimens from each of three consecutive stools using Hemoccult II® cards. Because specimen collection may be unpleasant and adversely affect compliance, a suggested solution is to advise the patient to dab a small amount of stool from the toilet paper directly onto the card.[6]
- Promptly return these three completed cards (six samples) to the laboratory.
- Test samples promptly. Approximately 14% of positive specimens become negative if left at room temperature for 2 days. A strong reaction will probably remain positive for at least 10 days. Rehydration with a drop of water before testing can increase the sensitivity up to 91%.[5]

3.   Evaluate the fecal occult blood test results.

One or more positive results in any of these six samples is considered to be a positive test for occult blood that cannot be ignored. After a race, marathon runners may have a positive fecal occult blood test.

---

*References 1,2,4,5,8,9.

†The diet should eliminate certain drugs (aspirin, nonsteroidal antiinflammatory agents, vitamin C, iron, laxatives), rare red meat, raw fruits and vegetables high in peroxidases (radish, horseradish, cantaloupe, cauliflower), and excessive amounts of foods moderately high in peroxidase (cucumber, carrots, grapefruit). Aspirin should be withheld at least 4 days before collecting specimens. Social consumption of ethanol (up to three bottles of beer per day or the equivalent) need not be restricted.[3]

In 1176 asymptomatic volunteers who were examined with both fecal occult blood testing and flexible sigmoidoscopy, neoplasia (adenomatous polyps or cancer) was found in 48 of those persons screened. Only 10 had positive stool occult blood, whereas 45 were detected by sigmoidoscopy. The fecal occult blood test detected only 18% of those screened with adenomas and 60% with invasive carcinoma. Flexible sigmoidoscopy detected 95% and 80%, respectively. Evaluation of the expected gain, by combining both tests, gave 18% for the fecal blood test and 94% for the endoscopic test.[10]

4.   If all fecal occult blood tests are negative, repeat the testing annually.

The American Cancer Society suggests that individuals at average risk after 50 years of age be initially screened with two sigmoidoscopy examinations and occult fecal blood testing done 1 year apart followed by annual examinations using occult fecal blood testing and digital rectal examination. Sigmoidoscopy should be done again every 3 to 5 years. Patients at higher risk should be screened more aggressively, for example, full colonoscopy every 3 years, perhaps supplemented by barium enema and flexible sigmoidoscopy.

5.   Evaluate every asymptomatic individual with a positive fecal occult blood test by either of the following approaches.

- Flexible sigmoidoscopy to 60 cm, plus air-contrast barium enema (if polyps are found by flexible sigmoidoscopy, perform full colonoscopy[1] instead of an air-contrast barium enema), *or*
- Full colonoscopy

Experts may evaluate the patient differently. The approach chosen may depend on the relative availability of skilled services.

With strict adherence to this testing strategy, about half of asymptomatic individuals with a positive fecal occult blood test will have significant colonic neoplasia—polyps over 5 mm will outnumber cancers (38% versus 12%). About 30% of these asymptomatic individuals with a positive fecal occult blood test will have benign sites of possible bleeding (polyps under 5 mm, diverticulosis, internal hemorrhoids); and 20% will have normal gastrointestinal studies.[1] Since it is possible that some of the 20% of individuals with normal gastrointestinal studies may have a lesion that was not detected, these individuals should be restudied in the near future, perhaps in a month or two.

A major drawback to improving the results of mass screening programs for colorectal cancer is the limited gastrointestinal workup conducted by physicians in many persons with a positive fecal occult blood test. In a screening program where 29,619 test kits were returned, 3.9% (1165) of the tests were positive. In 33% of persons with a positive screen, the diagnostic workup consisted of a repeated stool guaiac test and/or sigmoidoscopy only.[7]

6.   In patients with colorectal carcinoma, the following additional abnormal laboratory test results may occur.

HEMATOLOGY

- Decreased hemoglobin, hematocrit, or both, caused by iron deficiency anemia
- Leukocytosis caused by inflammatory complications of the tumor

- Increased platelets
- Increased erythrocyte sedimentation rate (ESR)

CHEMISTRY

- Hypokalemia with villous adenoma
- Increased lactate dehydrogenase (LD)
- Increased alkaline phosphatase (ALP); may produce Regan isoenzyme
- Hypoalbuminemia
- Increased carcinoembryonic antigen (CEA)

REFERENCES

1. Brendler SJ, Tolle SW: Fecal occult blood screening and evaluation for a positive test. West J Med 146:103, 1987.
2. Council on Scientific Affairs: Medical evaluations of healthy persons. JAMA 249:1626, 1983.
3. Fleming JL, Ahlquist DA, McGill DB, et al: Influence of aspirin and ethanol on fecal blood levels as determined by using the HemoQuant assay. Mayo Clinc Proc 62:159, 1987.
4. Frank JW: Occult-blood screening. Lancet 1:1204, 1986.
5. General Internal Medicine Subspeciality Committee: Medical Knowledge Self-Assessment Program. VIII. General Internal Medicine. Philadelphia, American College of Physicians, 1988, p 20.
6. Littenberg B: Stool collection for occult blood testing. Ann Intern Med 109:347, 1988.
7. McGarrity TJ, Long PA, Peiffer LP, et al: Results of a television-advertised public screening program for colorectal cancer. Arch Intern Med 149:140, 1989.
8. Questions about occult-blood screening for cancer. Lancet 1:22, 1986.
9. Ross CC: Screening for colorectal cancer. AFP 38:105, 1988.
10. Rozen P, Ron E, Fireman Z, et al: The relative value of fecal occult blood tests and flexible sigmoidoscopy in screening for large bowel neoplasia. Cancer 60:2553, 1987.
11. Urban E: Black stools (carcinoma of the cecum). In Cutler P: Problem Solving in Clinical Medicine: From Data to Diagnosis, 2nd ed. Baltimore, Williams & Wilkins, 1985, p 392.

DIGITAL RECTAL EXAMINATION AND PROSTATIC CANCER*

Carcinoma of the prostate is rare in the fourth decade, but the prevalence rapidly increases with age from 10% in the fifth decade to 50% in men over 80 years of age. It is the most common malignant tumor in elderly men. Only a small fraction of these cases becomes clinically apparent. There were 90,000 new cases and 24,000 deaths in 1986 in the United States. The strategy for detecting carcinoma of the prostate centers on digital rectal examination of the gland. All other tests and procedures are ancillary to this important part of the physical examination. Transrectal ultrasonic prostate imaging for detecting prostatic carcinoma is promising, but there are no clinical studies that convincingly support prostatic ultrasound as a superior diagnostic screen for prostatic cancer. Although ultrasound may be more sensitive than digital examination, it is less specific. Currently, it is most useful for defining extent of a known cancer

---

*Includes discussion of acid phosphatase and prostate-specific antigen.

with respect to the presence or absence of capsular penetration. Serum prostate-specific antigen (PSA) is more sensitive for prostatic cancer than is prostatic acid phosphatase (PAP); however, like acid phosphatase, it is not completely specific. It is more useful for determining adequacy of surgery for prostatic cancer or recurrence of prostatic cancer than for initially screening for or diagnosing prostatic cancer.[2,8,9,11,12,I]

1. Perform an annual digital rectal examination of the prostate to discover induration or nodular irregularities in men 40 years of age to detect carcinoma of the prostate.

Digital rectal examination is the most accurate and economical way to detect carcinoma of the prostate. It is more sensitive than measurement of serum PAP by any method. In a group of 300 men examined by urologists in which the prevalence of cancer was 23%, rectal digital examination had a sensitivity of 69%, a specificity of 89%, a positive predictive value of 67%, and a negative predictive value of 91%.[7,11] The American Cancer Society recommends that after 40 years of age men should undergo a digital rectal examination annually.

2. If a digital rectal examination of the prostate reveals an area of nodularity or induration, establish the diagnosis by obtaining a biopsy. Draw a blood specimen for PAP and PSA before the biopsy.

A needle-core biopsy of a prostatic nodule is the best way to document prostatic carcinoma. Prostatic biopsy may elevate PAP and PSA. Fine-needle aspiration has been gaining increasing popularity for the diagnosis of prostate cancer.[11]

3. If the diagnosis of carcinoma is confirmed histologically, review the serum PAP and PSA. Other helpful tests include a complete blood count (CBC), urinalysis, serum urea nitrogen, creatinine, alkaline phosphatase (ALP), lactate dehydrogenase (LD), and liver function tests.

Once the diagnosis has been established, it is important to determine whether the tumor is confined to the prostate or spread beyond the gland. This can be accomplished by a combination of laboratory tests and radiographic procedures.

Although serum PAP is rarely elevated when the carcinoma is confined to the gland, approximately 80% of patients with locally invasive or metastatic carcinoma will have sustained elevations. In addition to prostatic cancer, serum PAP may be elevated secondary to prostatitis, prostatic infarct, prostatic surgery or biopsy, Gaucher's disease, Niemann-Pick disease, some benign and malignant hematologic disorders, and other miscellaneous conditions.[10]

Although prostatic massage may elevate serum PAP for 72 hours, routine digital examination appears to have no effect.[3] Levels are raised in 9% to 55% of patients with benign hyperplasia, prostatitis, or retention of urine. It is not possible to determine whether such patients also have subclinical carcinoma of the prostate.

The serum PSA may be elevated twofold with prostatic massage, fourfold with cystoscopy, and more than fiftyfold with needle biopsy or transurethral resection of the prostate. Since the effective half-life of PSA is more than 2 days.

a needle biopsy would require a delay of 12 days before a measurement of PSA would be valid.[5,13] In another study, digital rectal examination had no effect on either PAP or PSA.[1]

PAP is rapidly destroyed at room temperature. The blood sample should be drawn without hemolysis and the serum rapidly separated from the cells. Either assay the serum immediately or freeze it until the time of analysis.

Tests other than serum PAP and PSA can detect secondary effects of the tumor. Serum ALP can be elevated because of osteoblastic bone metastases or cholestatic liver metastases. These ALP elevations may occur in individuals who have an elevated or normal PAP. In patients with metastatic carcinoma who have a normal PAP, an elevated ALP may alert you to the presence of metastatic disease and a CBC can detect secondary anemia. Serum urea nitrogen, creatinine, and urinalysis can detect renal dysfunction, such as an obstructive uropathy. Serum LD, specifically LD-5, may be elevated secondary to the tumor mass. It is wise to measure baseline PSA, since this will be useful for comparing future measurements of PSA to determine adequacy of surgical removal of the cancer or recurrence.

4.   If the needle biopsy of the prostate is negative for carcinoma, the patient is probably free of disease, but remember that false-negative biopsy and test results may occur.

About 50% of prostatic nodules felt on rectal examination will prove to be carcinoma. A single needle biopsy has a sensitivity to detect the carcinoma of about 80%, and the sensitivity increases to about 90% with repeated attempts.

The serum PAP is rarely elevated if the carcinoma is confined to the prostate gland, but about 80% of patients with carcinoma outside the gland, either soft tissue or bony metastatic disease, will have sustained elevations. False-negative results are more likely to occur in patients with poorly differentiated metastatic cancer.

Up to 90% of patients with prostatic carcinoma metastatic to bone will have an elevated serum ALP because of osteoblastic activity. Liver metastases can also cause an elevation of ALP that is secondary to cholestasis.

A negative chemistry and hematology screen—including a negative serum PAP—does not completely rule out prostatic carcinoma.[1]

5.   Evaluate the tests.

The best chemical methods for measuring serum PAP are the tartrate-inhibited fraction using p-nitrophenylphosphate or, more recently, using thymolphthalein monophosphate. An immunoassay for PAP may be substituted for a colorimetric assay. An immunoassay for PSA should be provided. Use the reference ranges for the assays provided by your laboratory.[4]

6.   Stage the tumor using test results in the context of clinical findings and radiographic data.

Prostatic carcinoma is staged by a combination of clinical findings, histology, laboratory test results, and radiographic findings. A standard scheme is the Whitmore-Jewett system, which stages the tumor according to tumor volume

REFERENCE RANGE VALUES[14]

TEST	SPECIMEN	REFERENCE RANGE (CONVENTIONAL)	REFERENCE RANGE (INTERNATIONAL)
Acid phosphatase: *p*-Nitrophenyl- phosphate	Serum	*Total* M*: 2.5–11.7 U/L F†: 0.3–9.2 U/L	2.5–11.7 U/L 0.3–9.2 U/L
		Tartrate-inhibited fraction M: 0.2–3.5 U/L F: 0–0.8 U/L	0.2–3.5 U/L 0–0.8 U/L
Acid phosphatase: Thymolphthalein monophosphate	Serum, ACA‡	<0.8 U/L	<0.8 U/L
Prostate-specific antigen	Serum§	0–4.3 ng/ml	

*Male.
†Female.
‡Automatic Clinical Analyzer (EI du Pont de Nemours & Co., Inc., Wilmington).
§Tandem®-R PSA (Hybritech, Inc., San Diego).

and whether it is still within the gland (focal or diffuse), extended beyond the gland, or widespread (pelvic lymph nodes or metastases). Bone marrow aspiration, which was used in the past to search for occult metastatic disease, is not indicated in the presence of a normal bone scan and should be reserved for evaluation of equivocal lesions.[11]

7. In addition to standard clinical procedures, including PAP and ALP, monitor the response of prostatic carcinoma to treatment using PSA.

PSA should be the standard marker for evaluating the response of prostatic carcinoma to treatment; it reflects the clinical activity of the disease in 97% of patients, especially when PAP levels, Gleason histologic grade, and clinical stage are taken into account. Raised PSA levels may precede the development of clinically detectable metastases by as much as 6 to 12 months.[6,12]

8. In men with prostatic carcinoma, the following additional abnormal laboratory test results may occur.

HEMATOLOGY

• Decreased hemoglobin, hematocrit, or both
• Elevated monocytes

CHEMISTRY

• Hyperglycemia
• Elevated creatinine and urea nitrogen
• Elevated uric acid

- Hypercalcemia with metastases to bone
- Hypophosphatemia

- Elevated aspartate aminotransferase (AST or SGOT)
- Elevated lactate dehydrogenase (LD)
- Elevated gamma-glutamyl transferase (GGT)

- Hypoalbuminemia

- Elevated carcinoembryonic antigen (CEA)

REFERENCES

1. Brawer MK, Schifman RB, Ahmann FR, et al: The effect of digital examination on serum levels of prostate-specific antigen. Arch Pathol Lab Med 112:1110, 1988.
2. Cutler P: Weakness, weight loss, anorexia (prostatic cancer). In Cutler P: Problem Solving in Clinical Medicine: From Data to Diagnosis, 2nd ed. Baltimore, Williams & Wilkins, 1985, p 523.
3. Daar AS, Merrill CR, Moolla SM, et al: Rectal examination and acid phosphatase: evidence for a persistence of a myth. Br Med J 282:1378, 1981.
4. Gambino R: Prostatic acid phosphatase and prostate-specific antigen: Immunoassays should replace colorimetric assays. Lab Rep Phys 11:9, 1989.
5. Gittes RF: Prostate-specific antigen. N Engl J Med 317:954, 1987.
6. Guinan P, Bhatti R, Ray P: An evaluation of prostate specific antigen in prostatic cancer. J Urol 137:686, 1987.
7. Guinan P, Bush I, Ray V, et al: The accuracy of the rectal examination in the diagnosis of prostate carcinoma. N Engl J Med 303:499, 1980.
8. Koss LG: The puzzle of prostatic carcinoma. Mayo Clin Proc 63:193, 1988.
9. Lee F, Littrup PJ, Torp-Pedersen ST, et al: Prostatic cancer: Comparison of transrectal ultrasound and digital rectal examination for screening. Radiology 168:389, 1988.
10. Lott JA, Wolf PL: Clinical Enzymology: A Case Oriented Approach. New York, Field, Rich and Assoc Inc, 1986, p 27.
11. O'Brien WM, Lynch JH: Current approaches to prostate cancer. Hosp Pract 23:143, 1988.
12. Prostate-specific antigen. Lancet 2:318, 1988.
13. Stamey TA, Yang N, Hay AR, et al: Prostate-specific antigen as a serum marker for adenocarcinoma of the prostate. N Engl J Med 317:909, 1987.
14. Tietz NW (ed): Clinical Guide to Laboratory Tests. WB Saunders Co, Philadelphia, 1983, p 8.

CHAPTER 2

ACQUIRED IMMUNODEFICIENCY SYNDROME (AIDS)

EARLY DETECTION OF ALCOHOLISM

URINE SCREENING FOR DRUG ABUSE

GENERAL AND MISCELLANEOUS PROBLEMS

ACQUIRED IMMUNODEFICIENCY SYNDROME (AIDS)

The acquired immunodeficiency syndrome (AIDS) is a clinical disorder resulting from infection with the human immunodeficiency virus (HIV), a retrovirus, in which the patient exhibits severe immunodeficiency and a rapidly progressive course characterized by opportunistic infections and neoplasms. Other outcomes of HIV infection include an asymptomatic carrier state and a disorder in which there is generalized lymphadenopathy that may be symptomatic, the AIDS-related complex (ARC). Since the first report of AIDS in 1981, more than 60,000 cases have been reported in the United States; 20,745 cases were reported in 1987 alone, a 57% increase over the number reported in 1986, and at least 30,000 additional cases have been reported from other countries. In the United States there are an estimated 1 million to 2 million individuals infected with HIV. The diagnosis of AIDS and ARC relies on the demonstration of HIV antibodies and other tests of compromised immunity together with the appropriate clinical findings. These findings include evidence of opportunistic infections and neoplasm. The mortality associated with AIDS exceeds 80% within 3 years of diagnosis, and the mean time from diagnosis of AIDS to death is less than 2 years.[8,V]

1. In patients with clinical findings of ARC or AIDS or if you wish to screen for infection with HIV, request an enzyme-linked immunoassay (ELISA) for HIV antibodies and confirm positive test results with a Western blot analysis, which identifies antibodies to specific viral proteins. Remember that ARC and AIDS are primarily clinical diagnoses and that HIV testing has significant legal, ethical, sociologic, and emotional implications.*

Even though disorders associated with HIV infection are primarily clinical diagnoses, in some settings, such as donating blood or belonging to the armed forces, a screening test for serum HIV antibodies is done in asymptomatic individuals. Because the prevalence of true HIV infection is very low in these asymptomatic individuals, false-positive test results are more likely to occur than when symptomatic individuals and individuals with positive risk factors are tested. The antibody titer can be helpful in identifying true-positive cases.

*Appropriate considerations for hospital policies on HIV testing follow: (1) the testing must support a defined goal for the health of the patient, his or her contacts, or the public health; (2) the patient must be informed and testing consented to by the patient; (3) testing must always be accompanied by counseling and guidance; (4) health and hospital care must not be in any way conditional on consenting to be tested or the results of the test; and (5) the confidentiality of test results must be maintained.[5,11]

More than 90% of individuals with AIDS harbor antibodies to the virus, and more than 95% of asymptomatic carriers of the virus are antibody positive. Currently available ELISA tests appear to have a false-positive rate of much less than 1% and a false-negative rate of less than 3%. In contrast, cultures of HIV have a high false-negative rate (30% to 70%). Therefore cultures have little role in the routine evaluation of patients.[V]

ARC can be diagnosed when an individual infected with HIV demonstrates persistent clinical abnormalities that fall short of the definition of AIDS. These include fever, weight loss, generalized lymphenadenopathy, diarrhea, fatigue, and night sweats. Appropriate laboratory tests include a complete blood count (CBC), serum protein electrophoresis, serum immunoglobulins, lymphocyte count, T helper cells, ratio of T helper to suppressor cells, and serologic tests for Epstein-Barr virus, cytomegalovirus, herpes virus, and hepatitis B virus.[9]

AIDS can be diagnosed when an individual infected with HIV demonstrates opportunistic infection or neoplasm in addition to appropriate laboratory test abnormalities. Infections include *Pneumocystis carinii* pneumonia; *Toxoplasma gondii* infection of the central nervous system; diarrhea caused by *Cryptosporidium* infection; strongyloidiasis; oral candidiasis; cryptococcal meningitis; other fungal infections (histoplasmosis, coccidioidomycosis, aspergillosis); mycobacterial infections; bacterial infections such as *Nocardia*, *Legionella*, *Salmonella*, *Shigella*, *Campylobacter jejuni*, and syphilis; viral infections such as herpes simplex virus, cytomegalovirus, viral hepatitis, Epstein-Barr virus, and progressive multifocal leukoencephalopathy (papovavirus). Neoplasms include Kaposi's sarcoma, epithelioid angiomatosis, non-Hodgkin's lymphoma, and Hodgkin's disease. Appropriate laboratory studies to obtain are the same as for ARC plus additional studies necessary to diagnose opportunistic infection and neoplasm. In patients with neuropsychiatric findings (at least 60%), consider obtaining cerebrospinal fluid for routine studies and viral culture (if available).[V]

Systems for classifying or staging HIV infections are available that rely on clinical and laboratory findings. In these systems, individuals may be categorized according to whether they have a recent infection, an asymptomatic infection, an infection characterized by lymphadenopathy, or an infection complicated by other diseases. Laboratory tests, such as HIV viremia, p24 antigen, p24 antibody, CD4 cell number, and beta 2 microglobulin, may also be used.[2,8]

2. Evaluate the tests.

Currently, HIV infection is detected by a positive ELISA test and confirmed by a positive Western blot analysis. If the ELISA antibody titer is high, it is more likely to represent a true-positive result than if it is low. The great disadvantage of the Western blot test is the lack of standardization of reagents, test methods, and test-interpretation criteria. The Western blot test should only be performed in laboratories with adequate proficiency. To maintain skill levels, testing should be done at least weekly, appropriate controls should be used, and the laboratory should participate in a regular, vigorous, external proficiency-testing program. Because of the subjective nature of interpretations, results should be reviewed independently by at least two laboratory specialists, one of whom is at the supervisory or director level.[3,4,10,12]

A new 5-minute HIV antibody test was recently approved by the Food and

Drug Administration. Early studies indicate that this test is quite accurate in the hands of well-trained laboratory technologists; however, when used by non-laboratory health-care workers, the test may produce a large number of false-positive results.[6]

3. If the ELISA test and Western blot analysis are positive, consider the patient to be infected with HIV. Do not diagnose HIV infection solely on the basis of a positive ELISA test.

The specificity of the ELISA test may vary, and when persons come from a clinical class with a low prevalence of HIV infection, false-positive results are more likely to occur. To exclude false-positive results, every positive ELISA test should be confirmed by a Western blot analysis. Western blot tests can be difficult to interpret, and many sera cannot be classified as positive or negative and must be characterized as indeterminate. Since the concentration of HIV antibodies generally rises after their first appearance, indeterminate Western blot tests should be repeated every month.

Some false-positive results with current ELISA test kits occur because patients' sera can react with test components other than HIV antigens. For example, false-positive results may occur in patients with chronic liver disease, myeloma, and autoimmune disease. Currently, the Western blot test is the best method to eliminate these false-positive results.[12]

Culture for HIV is difficult. A new test, which can detect viral DNA in peripheral blood mononuclear cells, may prove to be a definitive confirmatory test as well as a method to diagnose HIV infection in patients without antibodies. This test, a selective DNA-amplification technique, is called the polymerase chain reaction (PCR). At present, however, it is not widely available.[8]

4. If the ELISA test is negative, conclude that the patient is probably, but not necessarily, free of HIV infection.

With the ELISA test, occasional persons infected with HIV will be negative for the antibody. Further, there is a period of 1 to 3 months during a primary HIV infection when an HIV-infected person is seronegative. Interestingly, some of these patients may have an acute febrile illness resembling influenza or infectious mononucleosis. The typical pattern of seroconversion is not universal, and prolonged periods of viral infection may occur in the presence of a negative ELISA antibody test. When the suspicion for infection is high, the ELISA test should be repeated periodically for at least 1 year.[8]

Patients with a variety of other diseases may have "AIDS-like" clinical findings, including abnormal laboratory test results, such as depressed helper/suppressor T cell ratios and polyclonal gammopathy. Do not automatically conclude that these patients have ARC or AIDS, particularly if they are seronegative, since these patients probably do not have ARC or AIDS.[7]

5. In patients with HIV infection, consider obtaining serial measurements of circulating CD4 cells and anti p24 as laboratory markers of prognosis.

Individuals with HIV infection who have the most extensive or rapid fall in the levels of CD4 (helper) lymphocytes or a falling absolute lymphocyte count are likely to have a worsening clinical condition. Likewise, in HIV positive individuals who are positive for both p24 and gp41 antibodies, subsequent loss of anti p24 heralds a worsening clinical condition.[9]

6. In patients with HIV infection, the following abnormal laboratory test results may occur:

HEMATOLOGY

- Normochromic, normocytic anemia common; occasionally, autoimmune hemolytic anemia
  Leukopenia, lymphopenia
- Thrombocytopenia, either immunologic thrombocytopenic purpura or thrombotic thrombocytopenic purpura

CHEMISTRY[1]

- Hypoglycemia related to pentamidine therapy, inanition, or sepsis
- Hypocalcemia associated with systemic illness or hypomagnesemia
- Cortisone and aldosterone deficiency secondary to opportunistic infection or ketoconazole
- Syndrome of inappropriate antidiuretic hormone caused by pulmonary or central nervous system infection or drugs
- Euthyroid sick syndrome caused by systemic illness
- Hypogonadism related to hypothalamic deficiency secondary to systemic illness or ketoconazole

IMMUNOLOGY

- Depressed helper T lymphocytes
- Depressed helper/suppressor ratio
- Hypergammaglobulinemia (IgG, IgA, IgM, IgD)
- Depressed blastogenesis (PHA or con A)
- Decreased or absent tests for delayed cutaneous hypersensitivity

7. In patients with HIV infection with neurologic disorders, the following cerebrospinal fluid test results mav be found:

- Mild lymphocytic pleocytosis
- Elevated protein
- Normal glucose

REFERENCES

1. Aron DC: Endocrine complications of the acquired immunodeficiency syndrome. Arch Intern Med 149:330, 1989.
2. Classification system for human T-lymphocyte virus type III/lymphadenopathy-associated virus infections. MMWR 35:334, 1986.
3. The Consortium for Retrovirus Serology Standardization: Serological diagnosis of human immunodeficiency virus infection by Western blot testing. JAMA 260:674, 1988.
4. Diagnostic tests for AIDS. The Medical Letter 30:73, 1988.
5. Eickhoff TC: Hospital policies on HIV testing. JAMA 259:1861, 1988.
6. Fast AIDS test may be hard for some users. *Wall Street Journal*, February 8, 1989, p B1.

7. Hollander H, Cortland DD: Misdiagnoses of common medical problems in patients referred to an AIDS clinic—"Pseudo-AIDS." West J Med 144:373, 1986.
8. Miles SA: Diagnosis and staging of HIV infection. AFP 38:248, 1988.
9. Neff J: Personal communication.
10. Schwartz JS, Dans PE, Kinosian BP: Human immunodeficiency virus test evaluation, performance, and use. Proposals to make good tests better. JAMA 259:2574, 1988.
11. Sherer R: Physician use of the HIV antibody test. The need for consent, counseling, confidentiality, and caution. JAMA 259:264, 1988.
12. Steckelberg JM, Cockerill FR: Serologic testing for human immunodeficiency virus antibodies. Mayo Clin Proc 63:373, 1988.

EARLY DETECTION OF ALCOHOLISM

In the United States, about two thirds of the population drink alcoholic beverages. Approximately 10 million are problem drinkers, and, of these, about 6 million are alcoholics. According to a new study, 10% of the drinkers consume half the total alcohol. After heart disease and cancer, alcoholism is America's third largest health problem. Nationwide, some 20% to 50% of all general hospital admissions may be alcohol related, and 15% of all office visits may be related to problems with alcohol, but only 2% to 3% are so diagnosed. There are four medical syndromes associated with alcohol abuse: (1) acute alcohol intoxication, (2) the acute alcohol withdrawal syndrome, (3) the chronic state of alcoholism, and (4) the medical complications of alcohol abuse. If the individual with alcohol abuse can be identified at the problem-drinker stage rather than the stage of advanced physical and social stigmata, recovery rates can run as high as 70% to 80% rather than 40% to 50%. Recently, it has been shown that physician intervention can reduce the number of individuals who drink excessively by about 20%.[18] The diagnosis of alcoholism depends on demonstrating an abnormal dependence on alcohol despite widespread adverse psychologic, physiologic, and socioeconomic effects. Certain abnormal laboratory test results can provide support for the diagnosis. Clinical findings include the acute effects of alcohol and the chronic organ damage that results from long-standing alcohol abuse. Recently, the adverse effects of alcohol on the cardiovascular system have been emphasized.[6,13]

1. If you want to detect individuals with alcoholism, ask the CAGE questions, The Brief Michigan Alcoholism Screening Test questions, and request appropriate laboratory tests.

When directly questioned about their drinking habits, individuals frequently underreport the quantity of alcohol they consume. The questions that follow detect alcoholism in a less confrontational way. Sometimes, individuals will deny drinking altogether. In this circumstance, laboratory test results and other clues, such as unexplained bruises and frequent ingestion of antacids for gastritis, become more important. A history of trauma can signal the presence of alcohol abuse.[16] Also, alcoholics often smoke and abuse other drugs.[5,V] Hypertension, cardiomyopathy, and cardiac arrhythmias are additional clues. Any patient with an odor of alcohol probably has a problem with alcohol.

The CAGE acronym focuses on Cutting down, Annoyance by criticism, Guilt feelings, and Eye-openers. The questions are as follows[2,5,7,8,12]:

1. Have you ever felt you ought to cut down on your drinking?
2. Have people annoyed you by criticizing your drinking?
3. Have you ever felt bad or guilty about your drinking?
4. Have you ever had a drink first thing in the morning to steady your nerves or get rid of a hangover (eye-opener)?

The Brief Michigan Alcoholism Test has the following questions (Y = a yes answer and N = a no answer. The number after Y or N = the number of points for that yes or no answer)[3,5,14]:

1. Do you feel you are a normal drinker?	YES	NO	N2
2. Do friends or relatives think you are a normal drinker?	YES	NO	N2
3. Have you ever attended a meeting of Alcoholics Anonymous?	YES	NO	Y5
4. Have you ever lost friends, girlfriends, or boyfriends because of drinking?	YES	NO	Y2
5. Have you ever gotten into trouble at work because of drinking?	YES	NO	Y2
6. Have you ever neglected your obligations, your family, or your work for 2 or more days in a row because you were drinking?	YES	NO	Y2
7. Have you ever had delirium tremens (DTs), had severe shaking, heard voices, or seen things that weren't there after heavy drinking?	YES	NO	Y2
8. Have your ever gone to anyone for help about your drinking?	YES	NO	Y5
9. Have you ever been in a hospital because of drinking?	YES	NO	Y5
10. Have your ever been arrested for drunk driving or driving after drinking?	YES	NO	Y2

Laboratory tests that may be useful include a blood alcohol measurement; a complete blood count (CBC); erythrocyte indices, examination of a Wright-stained blood smear for macrocytic erythrocytes; and liver function tests including a serum gamma-glutamyl transferase (GGT). It may be worthwhile to obtain a biochemical profile and urinalysis, since so may analytes can be affected in alcoholism. Urinary alcohol determinations on daily samples collected for at least 1 week have also been recommended as an effective screening test for occult alcoholism.[9]

2. Evaluate the questionnaires and the laboratory tests.

Once ingested, ethanol is rapidly cleared from the blood, and after 24 hours it is completely gone. Changes in hematologic values, liver enzymes, and serum lipid levels persist for longer periods of time.

COMPARISON OF SENSITIVITY AND SPECIFICITY OF SCREENING TESTS FOR ALCOHOLISM*

TEST	SENSITIVITY (%)	SPECIFICITY (%)
CAGE (one question positive)	85	89
Mean corpuscular volume (MCV)	63	64
Gamma-glutamyl transferase (GGT)	54	76
Aspartate aminotransferase (AST or SGOT), alanine aminotransferase (ALT or SGPT), or alkaline phosphatase (ALP)	37	81

*Adapted from Bush B, Shaw S, Cleary P, et al: Screening for alcohol abuse using the CAGE questionnaire. Am J Med 82:231, 1987. Reprinted with permission.

BRIEF MICHIGAN ALCOHOLISM SCREENING TEST[5,14,15]

A score of 6 or more points indicates a probable diagnosis of alcoholism.

U.S. NATIONAL COUNCIL ON ALCOHOLISM (NCA) CRITERIA FOR ALCOHOLISM[4]

BLOOD ALCOHOL LEVEL	FINDINGS
>100 mg/dl (>22 mmol/L)	At the time of routine examination by a physician
>150 mg/dl (>33 mmol/L)	Without gross evidence of intoxication
>300 mg/dl (>66 mmol/L)	At any time

Although present laboratory tests lack diagnostic sensitivity and specificity, better tests may become available, for example, platelet monoamine oxidase and adenylate cyclase.[17]

3. If the answers to the CAGE questions, the Brief Michigan Alcoholism questions, and laboratory test results are consistent with alcoholism, the diagnosis is supported with a level of confidence that depends on the number of consistent answers and positive test results.

Even without laboratory tests, a history of heavy drinking, appropriate clinical findings, and consistent answers to the CAGE questions and Brief Michigan Alcoholism Screening questions may allow you to make the diagnosis. Of course, if laboratory test results are positive, they can lend considerable support to the diagnosis. A recent study showed that elderly alcoholics have more abnormal results of commonly used laboratory tests than do younger alcoholics. Interestingly, in this recent study, an elevated mean corpuscular hemoglobin (MCH) was the most sensitive test for the disorder in both elderly (71%) and younger alcoholics (57%).[10]

Although these questions and tests are quite sensitive for alcoholism, they are not completely specific. Occasionally, positive answers and test results will occur in patients who are not alcoholics. With the CAGE questions, three positive answers virtually eliminate nonalcoholics.[2] Also, there are other causes for an elevated GGT, such as therapy with phenytoin (Dilantin) or phenobarbital, and other causes for elevated transaminase and ALP levels, such as drug-related or viral hepatitis.

4. If the answers to the CAGE questions and the Brief Michigan Alcoholism Screening questions are negative and the laboratory test results are normal, the diagnosis of alcoholism is not supported by objective data.

Since the sensitivity of the CAGE questions and laboratory tests for alcoholism is less than 100%, negative answers and normal test results do not rule out the disorder with complete confidence. If clinical suspicion of alcoholism continues to exist, then the CAGE questions, the Brief Michigan Alcoholism Screening questions, and laboratory tests should be repeated in the future.

5. If you wish to monitor an alcoholic who is in a treatment program, measure GGT, AST (SGOT), and ALT (SGPT). If there is an odor of alcohol, measure blood alcohol.

When a patient is in a treatment program, a measurable level of blood alcohol provides evidence of failure to abstain from drinking. A more sensitive method to detect a drinking relapse is to measure GGT, AST (SGOT), and ALT (SGPT). An increase in any of these enzymes—GGT of 20% or greater, AST of 40% or greater, and ALT of 20% or greater—above an individual's values after 4 weeks of abstinence appears to indicate a return to drinking.[11]

6. In the alcoholic patient, additional abnormal laboratory test results may occur:

HEMATOLOGY

- Anemia caused by bone marrow suppression
- Leukocytosis caused by inflammation (e.g., of the liver or lung)
- Leukopenia from bone marrow suppression
- Thrombocytopenia from bone marrow suppression

CHEMISTRY

- Metabolic acidosis after severe alcoholic binge
- Hyperglycemia by interfering with peripheral glucose utilization
- Hypoglycemia in fasting patients because of suppression of gluconeogenesis by alcohol (As little as one or two drinks can cause this effect in any person.)
- Elevated uric acid (often >7 mg/dl [416 μmol/L])
- Hypokalemia
- Hypercalcemia following an alcoholic binge
- Hypocalcemia
- Hyperphosphatemia following an alcoholic binge
- Hypophosphatemia caused by poor diet, vomiting, diarrhea, antacids, and possible phosphaturic effect of alcohol, hypomagnesemia, and calcium deficiency
- Hypomagnesemia from dietary deficiency and increased urinary loss

- Elevated creatine kinase (CK) caused by myopathy, rarely myoglobinemia and myoglobinuria
- Elevated lactate dehydrogenase (LD) from myopathy
- Abnormal liver function tests caused by fatty liver, alcoholic hepatitis, or cirrhosis
- Elevated amylase in patients with acute pancreatitis

- Increased HDL-cholesterol, which returns to baseline after a week or two of abstinence
- Hypertriglyceridemia caused by increased hepatic production, often over 180 mg/dl (2.06 mmol/L)

- Modestly decreased thyroxine (T_4) and a marked decrease in serum triiodothyronine (T_3); return to normal after several weeks of abstinence
- Elevated cortisol following an alcoholic binge
- Decreased testosterone
- Inhibition of vasopressin secretion at rising alcohol concentrations and the opposite at falling concentrations, so that most alcoholics are often slightly overhydrated[II]

- Elevated serum osmotic pressure when measured by a freezing point osmometer but not a vapor pressure osmometer; provided other osmotically active substances, such as methanol or mannitol, are not present in the serum, the serum ethanol concentration can be calculated, based on the osmotic gap, as follows[VIII,7]:

$$\text{Estimated blood alcohol (mg/dl)} = \text{Osmotic gap} \times \frac{100}{22}$$

Where Osmotic gap = Measured osmolality − Calculated osmolality (all units in mOsm/kg)

Calculated osmolality (mOsm/kg) = 2 × Na (mEq/L) +

$$\frac{\text{Glucose (mg/dl)}}{18} + \frac{\text{Urea nitrogen (mg/dl)}}{2.8}$$

or

$$\text{Estimated blood alcohol (mmol/L)} = \text{Osmotic gap}$$

Where Osmotic gap = Measured osmolality − Calculated osmolality (all units in mOsm/kg)

Calculated osmolality (mOsm/kg) = 2 × Na (mmol/L) +
Glucose (mmol/L) + Urea nitrogen (mmol/L)

- Elevated carcinoembryonic antigen (CEA) in patients with alcoholic liver disease

REFERENCES

1. Bowen OR, Sammons JH: The alcohol-abusing patient: A challenge to the profession. JAMA 260:2267, 1988.
   Bush B, Shaw S, Cleary P, et al: Screening for alcohol abuse using the CAGE questionnaire. Am J Med 82:231, 1987.
   Cleary PD, Miller M, Bush BT, et al: Prevalence and recognition of alcohol abuse in a primary care population. Am J Med 85:466, 1988.

4. Criteria Committee, National Council on Alcoholism, New York: Criteria for the diagnosis of alcoholism. Ann Intern Med 77:249, 1972.
5. Crowley TJ: Alcoholism—Identification, evaluation, and early treatment. West J Med 140:461, 1984.
6. Cutler P: Strange behavior (alcoholism). In Cutler P: Problem Solving in Clinical Medicine: From Data to Diagnosis, 2nd ed. Baltimore, Williams & Wilkins, 1985, p 545.
7. Davis JE: Measurement of colligative properties. In Kaplan LA, Pesce AU: Clinical Chemistry. Theory, Analysis and Correlation. The CV Mosby Co, St. Louis, 1984, p 232.
8. Ewing JA: Detecting alcoholism. The CAGE questionnaire. JAMA 252:1905, 1984.
9. Gambino R: Biochemical profiles: Applications in ambulatory and preadmission testing of adults. In Glenn GC (ed): Blue Cross/Blue Shield Guidelines based on Common Diagnostic Tests. Use and Interpretation. Skokie, IL, College of American Pathologists, 1988, p. 20.
10. Hurt DH, Finlayson RE, Morse RM, et al: Alcoholism in elderly persons: Medical aspects and prognosis of 216 inpatients. Mayo Clin Proc 63:753, 1988.
11. Irwin M, Baird S, Smith TL, et al: Use of laboratory tests to monitor heavy drinking by alcoholic men discharged from a treatment program. Am J Psych 145:595, 1988.
12. Mayfield D, McLeod G, Hall P: More detailed interview screening. Am J Psych 131:1121, 1974.
13. Milhorn HT: The diagnosis of alcoholism. AFP 37:175, 1988.
14. Pokorny AP, Miller BA, Kaplan HB: A paper-and-pencil questionnaire. Am J Psych 129:342, 1972.
15. Screening for alcoholism. JAMA 260:476, 1988.
16. Skinner HA, Holt S, Schuller R, et al: Identification of alcohol abuse using laboratory tests and a history of trauma. Ann Intern Med 101:847, 1984.
17. Tabakoff B, Hoffman PL, Lee JM, et al: Differences in platelet enzyme activity between alcoholics and nonalcoholics. N Engl J Med 318:134, 1988.
18. Wallace P, Cutler S, Haines A: Randomized control trial of general practitioner intervention in patients with excessive alcohol consumption. Br Med J 297:663, 1988.

URINE SCREENING FOR DRUG ABUSE

Drug abuse (substance abuse) is a pattern of pathologic drug use for at least 1 month that leads to impairment of social or occupational functioning.[5] In the United States, its prevalence has reached epidemic proportions. For example, a 1983 survey revealed that 64% of young adults (18 to 25 years old) stated that they used marijuana, and a 1982 survey indicated that 22 million persons had tried cocaine at least once. Since 1986, use of crack, a potent and dangerous form of cocaine, has grown. Smoking crack can produce the same euphoric effect in users that intravenous injection does. Drug abuse is present in all socioeconomic groups, and its causes and origins are complex and poorly understood. A recent survey of employers indicated that 6% to 15% of their employees have an alcohol or drug problem.[10] The diagnosis relies on detecting the drug or drugs in the individual's body fluids—usually urine. Testing may occur in the context of a screening program or because of inappropriate behavior or drug-related illness. Documentation depends on laboratory tests. The clinical findings vary from relatively normal behavior to acute or chronic intoxication. There may be medical complications. Testing for anabolic steroids in athletes and bodybuilders is increasingly important, but only certain laboratories are capable of performing the analyses. Of twelfth-grade male students, 6.6% use or have used anabolic steroids.[1] Careful specimen collection and handling and reliable laboratory testing are critical.[8,II,V]

1. If an individual shows clinical findings of drug abuse, if you want to screen for drug abuse, or if you want to monitor a known drug abuser, obtain a urine specimen collected by a reliable observer, request appropriate tests, and maintain a chain of custody.* Consult your laboratory director or supervisor for information on anabolic steroid testing.

Blood is not a good specimen for drug abuse screening. The sensitivities of laboratory methods for detecting drugs in blood are not as good as in urine. Usually, the substances that can be detected in blood are limited to aspirin, acetaminophen, anticonvulsants, barbiturates, diazepam, and volatiles, such as ethanol.[3]

Clinical findings of drug abuse include mental changes (delirium, dementia, depression); school difficulties, behavior problems, or unexplained medical problems in adolescents or young adults; and a newly developing psychosis or unexpected deterioration in occupational or social functioning. Of course, known drug abusers should be tested to determine the specific substance or substances of abuse.

Screening for drug abuse is controversial. It is practiced by the federal government and many private industries. The value of workplace screening remains to be determined.

A critical issue in drug abuse testing is observation of collection of the urine specimen by a reliable observer to ensure that the specimen truly belongs to the subject being tested. Collection personnel can also inspect the urine color and measure its temperature, pH, and specific gravity, to verify specimen validity. The specimen should be accurately labeled and refrigerated, and a chain of custody should be maintained.

Appropriate tests for drug abuse should include those drugs most prevalent in the group or class to which the individual belongs. Screening by thin-layer chromatography is capable of detecting a wide spectrum of drugs. In contrast, screening by immunoassay will only detect the individual drugs that are included in the screening profile.

Because different drugs of abuse have different half-lives (e.g., cocaine: 40 to 80 minutes; amphetamines: 6 to 12 hours; marijuana or tetrahydrocannabinol [THC]: 4 to 6 weeks), different screening schedules are necessary to detect different drugs as follows.

2. Evaluate the tests.

Choose the most reputable laboratory available. You may wish to inquire concerning the laboratory's performance on outside proficiency surveys.[4,9]

Laboratories use two types of tests, screening and confirmatory, for detecting and confirming drugs in urine. Initially, a screening test is performed. A confirmatory test—using a more specific method—should be done to verify a positive screening test. The confirmatory test ought to be based on a different principle of analysis and be at least as sensitive as the screening test. Enzyme

---

*For drug test results to have legal validity, a chain of custody is required. This involves documentation of every person who had custody of the specimen from the time it was collected to the time it was tested. Moreover, every person who had custody must have kept the specimen in a secure manner, so that no one could tamper with it.[2,9]

DETECTION LIMITS FOR URINE DRUG TESTING*

DRUG	DOSE (MG)	DETECTION TIME	SCREENING FREQUENCY
Amphetamines	30	1–120 hr	1–2/wk
Barbiturates			
Short-acting	100	6–24 hr	1–2/wk
Phenobarbital	30	At least 4½ days	1–2/wk
Benzodiazepines			
Long-acting (diazepam)	10	7 days	1/wk
Short-acting (triazolam)	0.5	24 hr	2–3/wk
Cocaine	250	8–48 hr	2–3/wk
Methadone	40	7.5–56 hr	2–3/wk
Methaqualone	150	60 hr	1–2/wk
Morphine—opiates (IV)	10	84 hr	1/wk
THC metabolites	†	7–34 days	1/wk
	‡	6–81 days	1/mo

Source: Reprinted by permission of the Western Journal of Medicine, Saxon AJ, Calsyn DA, Haver VM, et al: Clinical evaluation and use of urine screening for drug abuse. West J Med 149:296, 1988.

*The detection time is the length of time that the drug can be detected in the urine after a given dose. The screening frequency is the suggested number of times per week or per month that urine drug testing would be required to detect repeated use of a given drug.

†Weekly marijuana use.

‡Daily marijuana use.

immunoassay (EIA), fluorescence polarization immunoassay (FPIA), and radio-immunoassay (RIA) are generally preferred for screening. Thin-layer chromatography (TLC) may also be used for screening. Gas chromatography (GC) and high-performance liquid chromatography (HPLC) are currently used for confirmatory analysis; however, gas chromatography–mass spectrometry (GC-MS) is the best confirmatory test.[2,7]

3. Interpret test results in the context of clinical findings.

As with all clinical laboratory tests, decisions must be made concerning what constitutes a positive test result. In marijuana screening, for example, establishing a threshold value of 100 ng/ml of urine will minimize the possibility of a positive result for persons with only a passive exposure to cannabis. Much lower levels can actually be detected. Using a higher threshold value of 100 ng/ml reduces the incidence of false-positive results but increases the incidence of false-negative results. A combination of enzyme immunoassay screening and GC-MS confirmation yields virtually 100% accuracy in detection of marijuana abuse.[6] The choice of a threshold value may be influenced by the clinical purpose of the test. The following table gives practical threshold concentrations for common drugs of abuse using different techniques.

THRESHOLD CONCENTRATIONS (IN μG/ML URINE)

DRUG	ENZYME IMMUNOASSAY	RADIO- IMMUNOASSAY*	THIN-LAYER CHROMATOGRAPHY[†]
Barbiturates	0.3–2.0	0.2–3.4	0.5–1.0
Amphetamines	0.3–1.0	1.0	0.3–0.5
Methadone	0.3	–	0.5
Benzodiazepines	0.3–2.0	0.1	1.0
Propoxyphene hydrochloride	0.3	–	0.5
Phencyclidine	0.08	0.025–0.10	0.1–0.2
Cocaine (benzoylecgonine- cocaine metabolite)	0.3	0.3	–
Opiates Morphine	0.3	0.3	0.25
Codeine	1.0	0.16	0.25
Cannabinoids (as total metabolites)	0.1	0.1	0.075–0.1
Methaqualone	0.3	0.75	1.0

Source: Reprinted by permission of the Western Journal of Medicine. Saxon AJ, Calsyn DA, Haver VM, et al: Clinical evaluation and use of urine screening for drug abuse. West J Med 149:296, 1988.

*Abuscreen® (Roche Diagnostic Systems, Montclair, NJ).

[†]"Traditional" thin-layer chromatography; sensitivity varies widely, depending on the system used.

Remember that, in contrast to ethanol, there is no established correlation between concentrations of drugs of abuse in body fluids and clinical impairment.

REFERENCES

1. Buckley WE, Yesalis III CE, Friedl KE, et al: Estimated prevalence of anabolic steroid use among male high school seniors. JAMA 260:3441, 1988.
2. Critical issues in urinalysis of abused substances: Report of the substance-abuse testing committee. Clin Chem 34:605, 1988.
3. Cutler P: Sudden coma (barbiturate intoxication). In Cutler P: Problem Solving in Clinical Medicine: From Data to Diagnosis, 2nd ed. Baltimore, Williams & Wilkins, 1985, p 536.
4. Davis KH, Hawks RL, Blanke RV: Assessment of laboratory quality in urine drug testing. A proficiency testing pilot study. JAMA 260:1749, 1988.
5. Diagnostic and Statistical Manual of Mental Disorders, 3rd ed. American Psychiatric Association, Washington, DC, 1980.
6. Moyer TP, Palmen MA, Johnson P, et al: Marijuana testing—how good is it? Mayo Clin Proc 62:413, 1987.
7. Peat MA: Analytical and technical aspects of testing for drug abuse: Confirmatory procedures. Clin Chem 34:471, 1988.
8. Saxon AJ, Calsyn DA, Haver VM, et al: Clinical evaluation and use of urine screening for drug abuse. West J Med 149:296, 1988.
9. Schwartz RH: Urine testing in the detection of drugs of abuse. Arch Intern Med 148:2407, 1988.
10. Workers Substance Abuse Is Increasing, Survey Says. New York Times, December 12, 1988, p 25.

CHAPTER 3

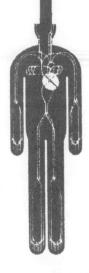

ANGINA PECTORIS AND ACUTE
MYOCARDIAL INFARCTION

CONGESTIVE HEART FAILURE

HYPERTENSION

CARDIOVASCULAR DISORDERS

ANGINA PECTORIS AND ACUTE MYOCARDIAL INFARCTION

Acute myocardial infarction (AMI) refers to sudden death of myocardial tissue secondary to coronary heart disease (CHD). According to the American Heart Association, 2.5 million Americans have angina and 1.5 million will have heart attacks in 1989. In 1987, about 978,500 Americans died from heart attacks, strokes, and other diseases of the heart and blood vessels. More men than women have infarcts, and the incidence increases with age. Although the electrocardiogram and, recently, radionuclide scintigraphic techniques are useful for the diagnosis of AMI, the best diagnostic tool is the detection of elevated blood levels of creatine kinase–MB (CK-MB) released from irreversibly damaged cardiac muscle fibers. The sensitivity of CK-MB for the diagnosis of AMI depends on how often we can detect an elevated blood level in the presence of AMI, and the specificity depends on how often the blood level is normal in the absence of AMI. In the future, tests for CK isoforms may detect AMI within 1 hour after onset. AMI can usually be recognized by its classical history and physical and electrocardiographic (ECG) findings; however, 10% to 20% of patients have silent or painless infarcts, and only about 60% to 70% of patients have characteristic ECG findings. Moreover, many patients with chest pains do not have CHD or AMI but have pain originating in the esophagus or pain caused by anxiety and other problems: up to 30% of those examined by coronary arteriography do not have CHD.[2,4,14]

1. In ambulatory patients with clinical findings of AMI, decide on hospital admission using the history, physical examination, and electrocardiogram. A serum CK/CK-MB can detect an unexpected AMI.

Hospital coronary-care units represent the standard level of care in the United States for patients who are thought to have an AMI. These coronary-care units are expensive, and it would be useful to be able to decide whether a given patient with clinical findings suggestive of AMI actually had an AMI before admitting the patient to such a unit. Because blood specimens are often drawn too early to detect the rise in enzymes, single measurements of CK and CK-MB isoenzymes in the emergency department are not sufficiently sensitive to exclude a diagnosis of AMI, and the decision to hospitalize the patient must be made on clinical and ECG findings. Using single test results in patients with chest pain in the emergency department, the CK was elevated in only 38% and the CK-MB in only 34%.[6,7] On the other hand, if the clinical findings do not suggest an AMI, a serum CK and CK-MB test can sometimes detect an AMI; however, false positives may be high. Because a single CK and CK-MB have low

43

sensitivity and specificity for AMI compared with serial samples, a 12- to 24-hour observation period with a second set of measurements may be useful in deciding whether to admit the patient.[7] *Silent or painless infarcts are more prevalent in diabetic patients and following cardiac transplantation.*[X]

Specimen collection and handling are important. An intramuscular injection can elevate total CK (not CK-MB) two to three times. Once the specimen is drawn, CK-MB starts to deteriorate within hours but with refrigeration is stable up to 24 hours. If more than 2 hours may pass before CK isoenzymes will be assayed, the serum sample should be preserved on ice.[6] CK-MB can be preserved for years with fast freezing, and lactate dehydrogenase (LD) will last for days at room temperature. Hemolysis interferes with LD measurements because erythrocytes contain 150 times more LD than serum, mainly LD_1.[VI]

2. In patients admitted to the hospital with clinical findings of AMI, request serial measurements of CK and CK isoenzymes. Serial measurements of LD and LD isoenzymes may be helpful. Serum transaminase measurements are unnecessary.

Although many clinicians measure serum CK and CK-MB more frequently, sampling at 0, 12, and 24 hours is adequate for diagnosis. Because some patients with AMI can exhibit a rise in CK-MB even though the total CK remains within the normal range, CK-MB should be measured. Failure to detect an elevated total CK may be caused by inadequate sampling.[18] The rise and subsequent fall of CK and CK-MB in AMI are characteristic. Commonly, LD and LD isoenzymes have been measured at 0 hours and every 24 hours for 2 to 3 days. Recently, it has been suggested that LD studies are confirmatory, are not always necessary, and may only be required if the patient's admission has been delayed more than 24 hours or if the CK studies fail to show an abnormality. If the serum total LD is normal, LD isoenzymes may not be needed.[13] If chest pain recurs after admission, a new set of CK and CK-MB measurements are indicated at 0, 12, and 24 hours.[6]

Serum CK rises within 3 hours of the onset of pain in a typical case of AMI. The peak level is reached about 24 hours later, followed by a decline to normal after another 48 to 72 hours. The duration of the rise and fall of the CK-MB fraction is similar to that of the total CK level. Serum LD rises in 8 to 12 hours, peaks in 48 to 72 hours, and becomes normal after 8 to 14 days. An elevated LD_1/LD_2 (over 1.0) usually appears in 12 to 24 hours, peaks in 48 hours, and is present in less than 50% of patients after 1 week.[1,VIII]

3. Evaluate the tests.

Some CK-MB assays are qualitative and measure only the presence or absence of CK-MB, whereas others are quantitative and express the CK-MB level in terms of its percentage of total CK with upper normal limits for CK-MB ranging from 3% to 6%. Electrophoretic methods for measuring CK-MB have been particularly satisfactory, giving good separation of isoenzymes and clinically reliable results. When compared with determination of CK-MB by electrophoresis, chemical methods for measuring CK-MB may give values that are more sensitive and less specific.

In the future, CK isoform analysis may enable us to detect AMI within 1 hour after onset. Earlier diagnosis of AMI will be be very helpful, such as in patients with equivocal clinical and ECG findings for whom thrombolytic therapy is under consideration. At present, rapid CK isoform tests are not generally available.[17]

A CK value of 1800 U/L or greater is most often seen in pathologic entities other than AMI, such as rhabdomyolysis, delirium tremens, and status epilepticus, and an LD value of 500 U/L or greater is most often seen in megaloblastic anemia, acute leukemia, metastatic carcinoma, trauma, and shock liver.[VII]

4. If the test results show a characteristic rise and subsequent fall of CK and CK-MB in the context of the appropriate clinical findings, conclude that the diagnosis is AMI. LD$_1$ and LD$_2$ elevations are confirmatory and, by themselves, can occur in other disorders.

An elevated serum CK-MB is the best method for diagnosing AMI, and in patients whose CK-MB levels are elevated within 24 hours of the onset of chest pain, the sensitivity approaches 100% and the specificity is very high. The rise and fall of CK-MB are characteristic. The sequence of an elevated serum CK-MB followed in time by an elevated serum LD with an elevated LD$_1$/LD$_2$ is unique for AMI. An elevated LD$_1$/LD$_2$ above 1.0 is 81% sensitive for AMI, and above 0.76 is 92% sensitive. The LD$_1$/LD$_2$ ratio may flip back and forth around 1.0 several times. Failure to detect an elevated LD$_1$/LD$_2$ in AMI may be related to inappropriate sampling times.[6] An isomorphic LD isoenzyme pattern (all isoenzyme values elevated) may indicate shock, an increased LD$_3$ may indicate pulmonary edema, and an increased LD$_5$ may indicate congestive heart failure.[16]

Suggested guidelines for enzymatic diagnosis of AMI include (1) serial elevation followed by a decrease in CK-MB to baseline with change of at least 25% between any two values; (2) increase of CK-MB of at least 50% between samples separated by 4 to 12 hours; (3) diagnosis of AMI, preferably made on at least two samples in a 24-hour period separated by at least 4 hours; (4) if only a single sample, elevation by at least twofold above normal; (5) diagnostic LD isoenzyme analysis if patient is admitted more than 72 hours from onset of infarction.[15]

The guidelines for interpreting serum CK/CK-MB test results for the diagnosis of AMI after noncardiac surgery are essentially the same as for the medical patient; however, after cardiac surgery, the guidelines are different. Surgical manipulation of the heart during cardiac surgery causes an elevation of CK/CK-MB at the time of surgery, which falls to normal over the next 12 to 18 hours. Persistent elevations after cardiac surgery suggest AMI.[6,10]

Numerous causes other than AMI can be responsible for an elevated CK/CK-MB. Cardiovascular causes include myocarditis, pericarditis, myocardial puncture or trauma, and acute dissection of the aorta. Systemic diseases with cardiac involvement can also cause elevations, such as muscular dystrophy, hypothermia, hyperthermia, and Reye's syndrome. Peripheral sources of elevations include myositis, rhabdomyolysis, athletic activity, prostate surgery, cesarean delivery, gastrointestinal surgery, and tumors. Miscellaneous causes include renal failure, subarachnoid hemorrhage, and hypothyroidism. An elevated LD$_1$/LD$_2$ without an elevated CK-MB can be found in hemolysis and renal infarction.[10]

Think of macro creatine kinase (macro CK) when the CK isoenzyme elevations do not fit the clinical picture. An autoantibody to CK-BB (macro CK, type 1) is a possible cause of macro CK, but macro CK may also be caused by release of mitochondrial CK into the serum (macro CK, type 2). Macro CK, type 1, is found in the sera of healthy persons and hospitalized persons, but macro CK, type 2, is found in severely ill persons of all ages, mainly those with various malignant tumors, including small cell carcinoma of the lung, cirrhosis of the liver, myocardial damage, and shock.[9,10,12]

5.   If serial measurements for elevated CK-MB and elevated LD_1/LD_2 are negative in a patient seen early after the onset of clinical findings of AMI, rule out AMI.

Serial measurements of CK, CK-MB, LD, and LD isoenzymes are also important for excluding AMI. If the levels are normal and no other significant disease is present, the patient can be discharged.

6.   In patients with AMI, estimate the infarct size by the degree of elevation of serum enzymes, but remember that the prognostic information may not be very good.

There is a relationship between the peak serum levels of CK, CK-MB, and LD and the size of an AMI with larger infarcts producing higher peaks. This relationship is stronger with CK and CK-MB than with LD. Infarct size can also be estimated from the time interval to peak CK, with longer times indicating larger infarcts. Frequent sampling, such as every 4 hours, is necessary to detect true enzyme peaks. Since there are a number of other variables, prognostic information is not very good. Routine measurements more often than 0, 12, and 24 hours are not indicated.[6]

7.   In patients with clinical findings of AMI, begin thrombolytic therapy as early as possible without waiting for enzyme and isoenzyme results. Measure serial levels of serum CK/CK-MB to monitor therapy.

Because the goal of thrombolytic therapy is to reopen an occluded artery as soon as possible, the decision to attempt thrombolysis should be based on clinical history and ECG rather than waiting for enzyme elevations. Ideally, in individuals without contraindications, thrombolytic agents should be used within 2 to 3 hours of the onset of findings. Waiting more than 4 to 6 hours is too long. About 60% to 70% of the treated individuals will have dissolution of the clot with reperfusion of the infarct about 1 to 2 hours after beginning therapy. Serum CK/CK-MB levels can be measured at 30-minute intervals for up to 2½ hours after initiation of therapy. Earlier and higher peak CK values have been observed in both spontaneous and iatrogenic reperfusion of an infarct. In successful thrombolytic therapy, CK increased an average of 34% (range of 13% to 67%) and CK-MB an average of 27% (range of 13% to 57%) in the first hour after reperfusion. This compares with an average CK increase of only 3% (range of 1% to 6%) and CK-MB of only 4% (range of 1% to 6%) in the last hour of a 2½-hour observation time in patients with unsuccessful therapy.[8]

8. In patients with AMI, additional abnormal laboratory test results may occur:

HEMATOLOGY

- Hematocrit may show a small early increase related to a decreased blood volume followed by a small later decrease.
- Leukocytosis, elevated erythrocyte sedimentation rate (ESR), and C-reactive protein caused by the inflammatory response associated with the infarct. Leukocytosis appears within hours of the onset of pain, persists for 3 to 7 days, and often reaches 12,000 to 15,000 leukocytes/mm³. The ESR rises more slowly, peaks during the first week, and sometimes remains elevated for 1 to 2 weeks.

CHEMISTRY

- Decreased pH with metabolic acidosis caused by tissue hypoxia.
- Decreased PO_2 from cardiopulmonary dysfunction. Mild hypoxemia can occur even without complications.
- Hyperglycemia related to diabetes mellitus as a predisposing risk factor or simply secondary to the stress of the infarct. In stress hyperglycemia, hemoglobin A_{1c} is normal.[11]
- Elevated urea nitrogen and creatinine related to decreased renal perfusion.
- Hyperuricemia.

- Hyponatremia.
- Hypokalemia caused by either a high level of circulating catecholamines or previous diuretic therapy. Hypokalemia may contribute to ventricular arrhythmia.

- Elevated aspartate aminotransferase (AST or SGOT) from infarct and possibly from hepatic congestion.
- Elevated alanine aminotransferase (ALT or SGPT) and LD_5 may occur from congestion and poor perfusion of the liver secondary to heart failure.

- Hypoalbuminemia caused by hepatic congestion.
- Hyperbilirubinemia with severe heart failure from hepatic dysfunction.
- Hypercholesterolemia, which may constitute a predisposing risk factor for coronary heart disease. If cholesterol can be measured within the first 24 hours, it is statistically the same as the preinfarction level.[3,5]
- Hypertriglyceridemia: peaks in 3 weeks and increase may persist for 1 year.

REFERENCES

1. Bakerman S: ABC's of Interpretive Laboratory Data, 2nd ed. Greenville NC, Interpretive Laboratory Data Inc, 1984, p 155.
2. Crawford MH: Substernal tightness (acute myocardial infarction). In Cutler P: Problem Solving in Clinical Medicine: From Data to Diagnosis, 2nd ed. Baltimore, Williams & Wilkins, 1985, p 306.
3. Gore JM, Goldberg RJ, Castelli WP: Cholesterol levels during acute myocardial infarction. Primary Cardiol 12(11):30, 1986.

4. Greenland P: Myocardial infarction. In Griner PF, Panzer RJ, Greenland P: Clinical Diagnosis and the Laboratory: Logical Strategies for Common Medical Problems. Chicago, Year Book Publishers, Inc, 1986, p 86.
5. Jackson R, Scragg R, Marshall R, et al: Changes in serum lipid concentrations during the first 24 hours after myocardial infarction. Br Med J 294:1588, 1987.
6. Lee TH, Goldman L: Serum enzyme assays in the diagnosis of acute myocardial infarction. Recommendation based on a quantitative analysis. In Sox HC (ed): Common Diagnostic Tests. Use and Interpretation. Philadelphia, American College of Physicians, 1987, p 19.
7. Lee TH, Weisberg MC, Cook F, et al: Evaluation of creatine kinase and creatine kinase-MB for diagnosing myocardial infarction: Clinical impact in the emergency room. Arch Intern Med 147:115, 1987.
8. Lewis BS, Ganz W, Laramee P, et al: Usefulness of a rapid initial increase in plasma creatine kinase activity as a marker of reperfusion during thrombolytic therapy for acute myocardial infarction. Am J Cardiol 62:20, 1988.
9. Litin SC, O'Brien JF, Pruett S, et al: Macroenzyme as a cause for unexplained elevation of aspartate aminotransferase. Mayo Clin Proc 62:681, 1987.
10. Lott JA, Wolf PL: Clinical Enzymology. A Case-Oriented Approach. New York, Field, Rich and Associates, Inc, 1986, p 149.
11. Madsen JK, Haunsoe S, Helquist S, et al: Prevalence of hyperglycemia and undiagnosed diabetes mellitus in patients with acute myocardial infarction. Acta Med Scand 220:329, 1986.
12. Martin LJ, Knight JA: Mitochondrial creatine kinase. Clinical Chemistry No. CC 88-10. Chicago, American Society of Clinical Pathologists, 1988.
13. Reis GJ, Kaufman HW, Horowitz GL, et al: Usefulness of lactate dehydrogenase and lactate dehydrogenase isoenzymes for diagnosis of acute myocardial infarction. Am J Cardiol 61:754, 1988.
14. Richter JE, Bradley LA, Castell DO: Esophageal chest pain: Current controversies in pathogenesis, diagnosis, and therapy. Ann Intern Med 110:66, 1989.
15. Roberts R: Enzymatic diagnosis of acute myocardial infarction. Chest 93(suppl): 3S, 1988.
16. Rotenberg Z, Weinberger I, Davidson E, et al: Atypical patterns of lactate dehydrogenase isoenzymes in acute myocardial infarction. Clin Chem 34:1096, 1988.
17. Wu AHB: Creatine kinase isoforms in ischemic heart disease. Clin Chem 35:7, 1989.
18. Yusuf S, Collins R, Lin L, et al: Significance of elevated MB isoenzyme with normal creatine kinase in acute myocardial infarction. Am J Cardiol 59:245, 1987.

CONGESTIVE HEART FAILURE

Congestive heart failure is a syndrome of passive congestion of the lungs, liver, and other tissues drained by the vena cava because of the inability of the heart to pump enough blood. In the United States its prevalence was recently estimated at 2.5 million. Heart failure can result from a cardiomyopathy, coronary artery disease, or some extramyocardial abnormality that interferes with cardiac filling or emptying, such as valvular heart disease, arrhythmia, hypertension, or constrictive pericarditis. Congestive heart failure can be diagnosed by a combination of clinical findings, electrocardiography, radiographic studies, and invasive techniques. The laboratory manifestations of congestive heart failure depend on the detection of secondary organ dysfunction caused by inadequate perfusion or passive congestion or both. Major organ systems affected include the lungs, liver, kidneys, and electrolyte homeostasis. It is useful to describe congestive heart failure in terms of left-sided failure and right-sided failure. In left-sided failure, the left atrial pressure is elevated and there are signs of pulmonary congestion. In right-sided failure, the right atrial pressure is elevated and there are signs of systemic venous hypertension and congestion. Clinical manifestations of congestive heart failure include dyspnea, orthopnea, pleural effusion, ascites, edema, and congestive hepatomegaly.[2,3]

1.   In patients with clinical findings of congestive heart failure, assess organ dysfunction by requesting serum electrolytes, urea nitrogen, creatinine, liver function tests, arterial blood gas levels, and a urinalysis.

Although serum electrolytes are generally normal before treatment, diuretic therapy and sodium restriction can cause abnormalities. Reductions in renal blood flow can increase serum urea nitrogen and creatinine concentrations, and congestion of the liver and kidneys can cause abnormal liver function test results and urinalysis findings, respectively. Congestion of the lungs can cause pulmonary edema and affect arterial blood gas levels.

2.   Interpret test results in the context of clinical findings.

Prolonged rigid sodium restriction coupled with intensive diuretic therapy, as well as the inability to excrete water, may lead to dilutional hyponatremia, which occurs despite an increase in total body sodium in the context of an expanded extracellular fluid volume. Prolonged administration of kaliuretic diuretics, such as the thiazides or loop diuretics, may cause hypokalemia. Recently, triamterene has been administered with thiazides for its potassium-sparing effect. In terminal heart failure, hyperkalemia may occur.[1]

The serum urea nitrogen, creatinine, and uric acid can be elevated secondary to reductions in renal blood flow and glomerular filtration rate. Urea nitrogen can increase as high as 80 to 100 mg/dl (13.3 to 16.7 mmol/L) and is disproportionately high relative to creatinine, that is, prerenal azotemia with an elevated BUN/creatinine ratio (normally about 10:1).

In right-sided failure, acute congestive hepatomegaly can cause significant elevations of serum transaminase (AST or SGOT and ALT or SGPT) levels to several thousand units, such that the findings resemble those of acute viral hepatitis. Low cardiac output is often present.[1] A differential clue is that, in contrast to viral hepatitis, the transaminase elevation of heart failure can be rapidly ameliorated by successful treatment. In acute myocardial infarction (AMI), the AST (SGOT) is elevated, but in AMI with congestive heart failure, both the AST (SGOT) and ALT (SGPT) are elevated. Other liver function tests can be abnormal, such as elevated serum alkaline phosphatase (ALP) and lactate dehydrogenase (specifically isoenzyme LD_5), as well as elevated total and conjugated bilirubin. In fact, frank jaundice can occur. The prothrombin time can be prolonged. Rarely, acute hepatic decompensation can occur, with hepatic coma and elevation of the blood ammonia.

A recent study categorized chronic congestive heart failure as mild, moderate, or severe. The mean values of all liver function tests in patients in the mild and moderate groups were essentially normal, except for minimally elevated alkaline phosphatase levels, slightly decreased albumin levels, and slightly increased gamma-glutamyl transferase (GGT) and bilirubin. In addition to these abnormalities, patients in the severe group had significantly higher levels of aspartate aminotransferase (AST or SGOT; 65 ± 82 U/L), alanine aminotransferase (ALT or

SGOT; 77 ± 102 U/L), lactate dehydrogenase (282 ± 91 U/L), and total bilirubin (1.7 ± 0.8 mg/dl [29 ± 14 μmol/L]).[4] In chronic congestive hepatomegaly, serum albumin can be decreased not only because of liver dysfunction but also because of a protein-losing enteropathy (a rare occurrence). Ascites is a late manifestation of heart failure.

In left-sided failure with acute pulmonary edema, arterial blood gas levels can be useful to assess oxygenation (decreased PO_2) with normal to decreased carbon dioxide (PCO_2).

Oliguria is characteristic of right-sided heart failure, and urinary specific gravity may be increased above 1.020.* During periods of diuresis, the specific gravity may be low. Mild albuminuria (<1 g/day) is common, and the urinary sediment may show isolated erythrocytes, leukocytes, and casts (hyaline and granular).

3. In patients with congestive heart failure receiving drug therapy, monitor the patient for possible adverse effects of drugs.

For example, thiazides and loop diuretics can cause alkalosis and decreased serum potassium, magnesium, glomerular filtration rate, and lithium clearance (in patients receiving lithium therapy), as well as increased serum glucose, uric acid, calcium, total cholesterol, LDL-cholesterol, triglycerides, and possibly plasma renin activity.[5] Uncommon effects include inappropriate antidiuretic hormone (ADH) secretion and decreased erythrocytes, leukocytes, and platelets.[V]

Potassium-sparing diuretics (triamterene) can cause megaloblastic anemia, increased potassium and plasma renin activity, and decreased glomerular filtration.[V]

To assess the effects of a drug on serum lipids, wait until the patient has been taking the drug for at least 6 to 8 weeks before measuring serum lipids.

In a recent study, serum electrolytes were measured in ambulatory patients with congestive heart failure at a median interval of 3 to 5 months.[3] The digoxin level was the next most common laboratory test.

4. In patients with congestive heart failure, the following additional abnormal laboratory test results may occur:

HEMATOLOGY

- Slightly decreased hematocrit even when red cell mass is increased
- Decreased ESR caused by decreased synthesis of fibrinogen secondary to congestion of the liver

CHEMISTRY

- Hyperglycemia common, probably related to stress
- Hypoglycemia possible with severe decrease in cardiac output and congestion of the liver

---

*In the setting of acute oliguria, the urine sodium concentration in congestive heart failure is generally below 20 mEq/L (20 mmol/L), whereas in acute renal failure or incomplete obstruction, the urine sodium is typically above 40 mEq/L (40 mmol/L).

- Hypomagnesemia caused by anorexia, malabsorption, and excessive use of diuretic agents[6]
- Hypocholesterolemia with severe congestion of the liver

REFERENCES

1. Cohen JA, Kaplan MM: Left-sided heart failure presenting as hepatitis. Gastroenterology 74:583, 1978.
2. Cutler P: Dyspnea on exertion (congestive heart failure). In Cutler P: Problem Solving in Clinical Medicine: From Data to Diagnosis. Baltimore, Williams & Wilkins, 1985, p 302.
3. Fleg JL, Hinton PC, Lakatta EG, et al: Physician utilization of laboratory procedures in outpatients with congestive heart failure. Arch Intern Med 149:393, 1989.
4. Kubo SH, Walter BA, John DHA: Liver function abnormalities in chronic heart failure. Influence of systemic hemodynamics. Arch Intern Med 147:1227, 1987.
5. Lardinois CK, Neuman SL: The effects of antihypertensive agents on serum lipids and lipoproteins. Arch Intern Med 148:1280, 1988.
6. Whang R: Magnesium deficiency: Pathogenesis, prevalence, and clinical implications. Am J Med 82(suppl 3A):24, 1987.

HYPERTENSION

The World Health Organization defines hypertension as follows: normal blood pressure is 139 mm Hg or less systolic and 89 mm Hg or less diastolic; high blood pressure is 160 mm Hg or greater systolic and 95 mm Hg or greater diastolic. For practical purposes, adult blood pressures of less than 140/90 can be considered as relatively normal, 140/90 to 160/95 as borderline elevated, and more than or equal to 160/95 as hypertensive. The important point is that risk for cardiovascular disease, heart failure, renal failure, and stroke increases progressively at levels above 130 mm Hg systolic and 85 mm Hg diastolic pressure. Hypertensive patients are at greatly increased risk of coronary heart disease (CHD)—they are two to three times as likely to die from myocardial infarction as from stroke. According to the American Heart Association, about 60 million Americans are hypertensive. The prevalence of hypertension is higher among blacks than whites, and it increases with age in all groups. Every patient with hypertension should have an evaluation (1) to provide baseline data for use in subsequent drug therapy, (2) to search for other risk factors, (3) to look for target organ damage, and (4) to find a specific cause. This evaluation should include a history and physical evaluation, an electrocardiogram (ECG), and certain laboratory tests. [1,2,5-7]

1. In patients with hypertension, request a complete blood count (CBC), serum glucose (fasting), urea nitrogen, creatinine, potassium, calcium, uric acid, cholesterol, HDL-cholesterol, and a urinalysis. Sometimes, these tests can be ordered as part of less costly batteries or profiles.

A hemoglobin and a hematocrit are useful to detect anemia, which can further stress the heart, and a baseline leukocyte count and platelet count may prove useful in monitoring drug therapy. An elevation of the fasting serum glucose can detect diabetes mellitus, which may be associated with accelerated atherosclerosis, renal vascular disease, and diabetic nephropathy; moreover, hyperglycemia can signal the presence of primary aldosteronism, Cushing's syndrome, and pheochromocytoma. Glucose levels may also be affected by therapy. Serum levels of urea nitrogen and creatinine, as well as a urinalysis, are useful to exclude renal parenchymal disease and to assess renal function. Serum potassium serves not only as a screen for mineralocorticoid-induced hypertension but also as a baseline before initiating drug therapy. Serum uric acid is affected by drugs and is often elevated in renal and essential hypertension. Hypercholesterolemia is another important risk factor for accelerated atherosclerosis, and serum cholesterol may be elevated by antihypertensive drugs, such as thiazide diuretics.[3,5,7]

2. Interpret test results in the context of clinical findings.

For most hypertensive patients, the laboratory evaluation, at this point, will be complete. Baseline data will be in place, and target organ damage will be assessed. Patients with an elevated cholesterol or low HDL-cholesterol should be studied further to determine LDL-cholesterol and triglyceride levels and whether the hypercholesterolemia is primary or secondary. Physicians may select additional tests based on their clinical judgment. Type and frequency of repeated laboratory tests should be based on the severity of target organ damage and the effects of the selected treatment program. If a specific form of secondary hypertension is suspected because of certain clinical and laboratory clues, commence studies for coarctation, Cushing's syndrome, pheochromocytoma, primary aldosteronism, and renovascular hypertension. Additional diagnostic testing should be reserved for cases in which potentially correctable causes of hypertension are suspected, including patients whose age at onset of hypertension is less than 30 years or more than 60 years and patients who respond poorly to aggressive medical management.[6,7]

3. In patients with hypertension receiving drug therapy, monitor the patient for possible adverse effects of drugs.

For example, beta blockers can cause increased serum potassium and triglycerides, as well as decreased HDL-cholesterol, glomerular filtration rate, and plasma renin activity.[3] A rare effect is a positive antinuclear antibody (ANA).[V] To assess the effects of a drug on serum lipids, wait until the patient has been taking the drug for at least 6 to 8 weeks before measuring lipid levels. Patients treated with antihypertensive drugs are at increased risk for diabetes. The time between the start of therapy and the onset of diabetes is about 8 years.[4]

REFERENCES

1. Caris TN: High blood pressure. In Cutler P: Problem Solving in Clinical Medicine: From Data to Diagnosis. Baltimore, Williams & Wilkins, 1985, p 531.
2. Coronary artery disease in hypertension. Lancet 2:1461, 1988.
3. Lardinois CK, Neuman SL: The effects of antihypertensive agents on serum lipids and lipoproteins. Arch Intern Med 148:1280, 1988.

4. Lundgren H, Björkman L, Keiding P, et al: Diabetes in patients with hypertension receiving pharmacological treatment. Br Med J 297:1512, 1988.
5. 1988 Joint National Committee: The 1988 report of the Joint National Committee on detection, evaluation, and treatment of high blood pressure. Arch Intern Med 148:1023, 1988.
6. Orland MJ, Saltman RJ (eds): Manual of Medical Therapeutics, 25th ed. Boston, Little, Brown & Co, 1986, p 57.
7. Gifford RW, Kirkendall W, O'Connor DT: Office evaluation of hypertension. A statement for health professionals by a writing group of the Council for High Blood Pressure Research, American Heart Association. Circulation 79:721, 1989.

CHAPTER 4

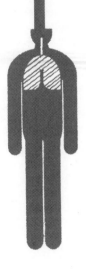

RESPIRATORY TRACT DISORDERS

ACUTE PHARYNGITIS

Acute pharyngitis has a variety of etiologies. The majority of these infections are caused by viruses for which antimicrobial drug therapy is not effective. Of the bacterial causes, group A streptococcal pharyngitis (between 5% and 15% of all cases of pharyngitis) has assumed major importance, because it may give rise to acute rheumatic fever (ARF) and acute glomerulonephritis (AGN). While ARF is less common in the United States than it was 30 years ago, it still persists and has recently surfaced in several regions of the country. The incidence of acute streptococcal pharyngitis is highest in children aged 5 to 15 years. Management of patients with acute pharyngitis relies on treating the patient with antibiotics when the probability of streptococcal pharyngitis is high and culturing when the probability is intermediate or low. It is important to keep other causes of acute pharyngitis in mind.[1-4,6,7,9]

1. In patients at high risk for streptococcal pharyngitis, treat with antibiotics without obtaining a throat culture or rapid diagnostic test. Groups at high risk (probably greater than 40%) include children over 3 years old and young adults with a combination of sore throat, exudate on the tonsils or tonsillar area, temperature greater than 37.8°C (100°F), and anterior cervical lymphadenitis (tender lymph nodes).
Withhold antibiotics and obtain a throat culture or rapid diagnostic test for group A streptococci in patients who have a sore throat but lack one or more findings of the high risk group. A Gram stain of exudative material may be helpful.
Leukocyte count, C-reactive protein, sedimentation rate, antistreptolysin O titer, and other laboratory tests are not helpful.

Other risk factors that increase the possibility of serious disease from streptococcal pharyngitis include immunosuppression and diabetes mellitus. A previous history of ARF, documented strep exposure, known strep epidemic, and a scarlatiniform rash are special risk factors.[4,I]

When the probability of group A streptococcal infection is greater than 40%, it is prudent to immediately treat the patient with antibiotics. Relying on throat culture or rapid diagnostic test results in this group would be inappropriate, since even in the best circumstances their sensitivity is only about 90%. Early treatment with antibiotics can prevent ARF and may also shorten the course of the illness, reducing fever and local and systemic symptoms.[2-4, 6-9]

On the other hand, when the probability of group A streptococcal infections is less than 40%, the risks of antibiotic therapy (drug reaction and fatal anaphylaxis) approximate the risks of acquiring rheumatic fever. Some experts advo-

55

cate dividing the patients not treated with antibiotics into a group at intermediate risk and a group at low risk for group A streptococcal infection and not culturing the low-risk group. However, in view of the resurgence of pockets of rheumatic fever in the United States, it may be wise to look for group A streptococcal infection in the low-risk group also.[1] A problem with treating a low-risk patient with a positive throat culture is that the throat culture may be falsely positive; that is, the patient may be a carrier.[4]

Consider the possibilities of mycoplasmal, gonococcal, or *Chlamydia trachomatis* pharyngitis in patients with persistent pharyngitis and a negative culture for group A streptococci or in patients with a positive culture who are not responding to penicillin. Consider infectious mononucleosis in patients with persistent systemic illness, lymphadenopathy, and splenomegaly. Consider diphtheria in unvaccinated populations, and look for a gray membrane that is firmly adherent to the tonsillar of pharyngeal mucosa. Specimens from both throat and nasopharynx should be submitted for culture confirmation of diphtheria.[4,9]

The most common and important respiratory viruses that can produce pharyngitis are rhinovirus, influenza virus, parainfluenza virus, adenovirus, the enteroviruses, cytomegalovirus, Epstein-Barr virus, and herpes simplex virus.[4]

2. Use good technique when obtaining the throat culture and use high-quality laboratory tests.

When obtaining the throat culture, using a Dacron swab (cotton fibers may inhibit *Neisseria*), vigorously rub the posterior pharynx, the tonsils or tonsillar pillars, and areas of purulence, exudation, or ulceration. A tongue blade will help prevent contamination with buccal organisms. Use of a self-contained collection/transport system, such as the Culturette® (Marion Scientific, Kansas City), makes collection and transport of throat cultures relatively simple and convenient. With good specimens and high-quality laboratory tests, the sensitivity for group A streptococci is about 90%. With poor specimens and poor-quality tests the sensitivity varies to as low as 29%. If you suspect gonococcal pharyngitis or the meningococcal carrier state, the swab is best inoculated onto a previously warmed JEMBEC plate (or other suitable medium) as soon as the culture is obtained. Inoculated plates should be incubated overnight at 35°C in an atmosphere of 5% to 10% CO_2 before shipment to a laboratory. Immediate shipment will result in killing of *Neisseria*, if present. Another option when *Neisseria* is suspected is to place the swab in a transport medium before sending it to the laboratory. Perform a test for heterophil antibody if you suspect infectious mononucleosis.

3. Evaluate the throat culture and rapid diagnostic test.

A positive throat culture or rapid diagnostic test for group A streptococci may reflect infection or an asymptomatic carrier state. In children, the carrier rate can be up to 15%.[9] At present, there is no accurate way to distinguish between true streptococcal infection and the carrier state at the time of initial presentation.[5] The false-negative rate of a well-performed single throat culture in infected patients is about 10%. Although the rapid diagnostic test is quite specific, it is not as sensitive as a culture: if negative in a patient at special risk, obtain a throat culture. A Gram stain of exudative material that shows Gram-positive cocci in chains is highly indicative of streptococcal infection.

4. If the throat culture or rapid diagnostic test is positive for group A streptococci, treat the patient with antibiotics.

Although streptococcal pharyngitis is a self-limited disease usually lasting less than 5 days, it appears that early treatment with antibiotics will significantly alleviate symptoms.[8] In areas where the incidence of rheumatic fever is rising, adequate antibiotic therapy will prevent this complication.[1] In immunosuppressed patients and diabetics, antibiotics may prevent serious disease.[4]

5. Perform follow-up cultures in patients who remain symptomatic, in patients who are at high risk for streptococcal sequelae, and in patients who live in close contact with those who are at high risk.

Do not perform routine follow-up cultures.

REFERENCES

1. Bisno AL, Shulman ST, Dajani AS: The rise and fall (and rise?) of rheumatic fever. JAMA 259:728, 1988.
2. Centor RM, Meier FA, Dalton HP: Throat cultures and rapid tests for diagnosis of group A streptococcal pharyngitis. Ann Intern Med 105:892, 1986.
3. DeNeef P: Selective testing for streptococcal pharyngitis in adults. J Fam Pract 25:347, 1987.
4. General Internal Medicine Subspecialty Committee: Medical Knowledge Self-Asssessment Program VIII. General Internal Medicine. Philadelpha, American College of Physicians, 1988, p 7.
5. Gerber MA, Randolph MF, Mayo DR: The group A streptococcal carrier state. Am J Dis Child 142:562, 1988.
6. Komaroff AL: Sore throat. In Lundberg GD (ed): Using the Clinical Laboratory in Medical Decision-Making. Chicago, American Society of Clinical Pathologists, 1983, p 133.
7. Komaroff AL: Sore throat in adult patients. In Griner PF, Panzer RJ, Greenland P: Clinical Diagnosis and the Laboratory: Logical Strategies for Common Medical Problems. Chicago, Year Book Medical Publishers, Inc, 1986, p 44.
8. Krober MS, Bass JW, Michels GN: Streptococcal pharyngitis. Placebo-controlled double-blind evaluation of clinical response to penicillin therapy. JAMA 253:1271, 1985.
9. Steinbrook R: Pharyngitis. West J Med 143:534, 1985.

ALLERGIC RHINITIS

Allergic rhinitis is a disorder characterized by sneezing, rhinorrhea, pruritus, and nasal obstruction, which usually lasts longer than 10 days and is caused by sensitivity to one or more allergens. It occurs in 7% to 10% of individuals between the ages of 11 and 50 years. Allergic rhinitis can be diagnosed by correlating the clinical findings with the presence of the offending allergen. Laboratory tests are ancillary to careful clinical observations.[1-4,7,9,10]

1. If the diagnosis of allergic rhinitis cannot be made from clinical findings, consider examining a nasal smear for eosinophils, measuring the

total serum IgE level, skin testing, and radioallergosorbent testing (RAST). The blood eosinophil count is not helpful.

The differential diagnosis of seasonal allergic rhinitis includes viral infection; abuse of nose drops and sprays; drugs, such as ovarian hormones, reserpine, hydralazine, and aspirin and other nonsteroidal antiinflammatory agents; and premenstrual or pregnancy-related hormonal rhinitis.[3,7,V]

The differential diagnosis of perennial allergic rhinitis includes nasal abnormalities such as deviated septum; endocrine abnormalities such as hypothyroidism, nasal mastocytosis, and idiopathic perennial nonallergic rhinitis (vasomotor rhinitis). Nasopharyngeal masses can mimic allergic symptoms.[3,7,8,V]

Nasal secretions should be examined for eosinophilia even if the blood eosinophil count is normal. The specimen may be collected as follows: blowing the nose onto waxed paper or cellophane, a swab in the nose for 2 or 3 minutes, or aspiration with a small rubber bulb syringe. The specimen is then transferred to a slide, dried, and stained with Wright's stain.[6] The blood eosinophil count is not useful, since it may be normal or increased in either allergic or nonallergic rhinitis. A positive test for nasal eosinophilia provides the same support for a diagnosis of allergic rhinitis as does an elevated total serum IgE level.

Skin tests are of value only in patients with clinical findings and should not be used for screening asymptomatic patients, since positive reactions will occur in many individuals who have no symptoms. In practice, skin tests are used to either advise patients concerning avoidance therapy or to help select antigens for use in therapy. Skin tests are the quickest and least expensive way to identify specific allergens.

RAST measures allergen-specific serum IgE antibody titers, and the results correlate well with skin testing. RAST is useful in patients where skin testing is inappropriate because of extensive eczema, marked dermatographism, or interfering medications.

2. Evaluate the tests.

A positive nasal smear in allergic rhinitis shows large numbers of eosinophils (usually more than 25% of all cells present).

A serum total IgE level that is low practically rules out atopy, whereas one that is high markedly increases the likelihood of this diagnosis.

RAST is said to be safer, more expensive, less sensitive, but perhaps more specific than skin testing; however, a recent study found the sensitivity and specificity of RAST and skin pricks to be almost identical.[5] Although RAST may give false-negative results, it rarely gives false-positive results. Unlike skin tests, it is not affected when the patient is taking antihistamine or sympathomimetic drugs.

3. If the test results are positive, they support the diagnosis, but the diagnosis must be made by considering the test results together with the clinical features.

A positive nasal smear for eosinophilia and an elevated serum total IgE support the diagnosis of allergic rhinitis but are not diagnostic. Eosinophils can also be found in the syndrome of nonallergic rhinitis with eosinophilia (NARES).[7]

Large numbers of neutrophils in the nasal smear suggest infection rather than allergic rhinitis. The manifestations of upper respiratory tract infection usually last no longer than a week and include fever, pain, and the presence of neutrophils in secretions.

4. If the test results are negative, do not necessarily conclude that the patient does not have allergic rhinitis or that the allergen tested is not responsible.

The tests for allergic rhinitis are not perfectly sensitive. For example, positive nasal smears for eosinophilia are found only in 50% of patients with proved allergic rhinitis, and the serum total IgE level is elevated in only 30% to 40% of patients with allergic rhinitis. Relief of symptoms by avoiding the suspected allergen is the best method of diagnosis.

REFERENCES

1. Council on Scientific Affairs. In vivo diagnostic testing and immunotherapy for allergy. Report I, Part I of the Allergy Panel. JAMA 258:1363, 1987.
2. Council on Scientific Affairs. In vivo diagnostic testing for allergy. Report II of the Allergy Panel. JAMA 258:1639, 1987.
3. Demichiei ME, Nelson L: Allergic rhinitis. AFP 37:251, 1988.
4. Druce HM, Kaliner MA: Allergic rhinitis. JAMA 259:260, 1988.
5. Ferguson AC, Murray AB: Predictive value of skin prick tests and radioallergosorbent tests for clinical allergy to dogs and cats. Can Med Assoc J 134:1365, 1986.
6. Ghory JE: Allergy of the upper respiratory tract and eyes. In Lawlor GJ, Fischer TJ (eds): Manual of Allergy and Immunology. Boston, Little Brown & Co, 1981, p 95.
7. Lieberman P: Rhinitis: Allergic and nonallergic. Hosp Pract 23:117, 1988.
8. Van Dellen RG, McDonald TJ: Nasopharyngeal masses mimicking "allergic" nasal symptoms. Mayo Clin Proc 63:69, 1988.
9. Van Ardsdel Jr. PP, Larson EB: Diagnostic tests for patients with suspected allergic disease. Utility and limitations. Ann Intern Med 110:304, 1989.
10. American College of Physicians: Allergy testing. Ann Intern Med 110:317, 1989.

COMMUNITY-ACQUIRED PNEUMONIA

Pneumonia is the sixth leading cause of death in the United States. About 65,000 Americans die of the disease annually, with people over 65 years of age accounting for three fourths of the cases. It has been estimated that 3.3 million persons are treated as outpatients and over 500,000 persons require hospitalization for the community-acquired pneumonias in the United States each year. These acute infections are either bacterial pneumonias or mycoplasmal, viral, or other "atypical" pneumonias. There has also been a rise in the otherwise rare *Pneumocystis* pneumonia in AIDS patients and others with poorly functioning immune systems. Fungal pneumonia can occur but is unusual. The diagnosis is made on the basis of clinical findings, radiographs, and laboratory tests. Symptoms and signs include cough, fever, tachypnea, and pain in the chest when coughing or breathing deeply. A productive cough with demonstrable bacteria on Gram stain suggests purulent bronchitis or bronchopneumonia. This discussion will focus on community-acquired pneumonia and will not cover hospital-acquired pneumonia.[3,10]

1. In patients with clinical findings of pneumonia, request a chest radiograph, complete blood count (CBC), and leukocyte differential count. If sputum is available, obtain a Gram stain and culture. If the clinical findings are severe enough to require hospitalization, consider obtaining two blood cultures and arterial blood gases.

Whereas a Gram stain and a culture of sputum are useful, a Gram stain and a culture of saliva are useless. The patient should thoroughly rinse his or her mouth with water several times, take some deep breaths and hold them several times, and then attempt to bring up sputum from deep in the bronchial tree. Inhalation of a warmed 3% to 10% saline aerosol may be helpful. Sputum can be distinguished from saliva by microscopically evaluating the specimen under low power. Greater than 25 neutrophils and less than 10 squamous epithelial cells per low-power field indicate a good sputum sample. No specimen containing more than 25 squamous epithelial cells per low-power field should even be cultured, because it represents heavy contamination by oropharyngeal secretions. A good Gram stain not only can identify common causes of community-acquired bacterial pneumonia but also can determine when no bacteria are present (i.e., a viral pneumonia). Moreover, the Gram stain can determine a good specimen for culture and may even obviate the need for a culture.[5,9]

Other techniques are available to examine sputum: digestion with 10% potassium hydroxide to identify fungi; immunologic techniques, such as the quellung reaction for *Streptococcus pneumoniae;* counterimmunoelectrophoresis to detect bacterial antigens, such as *S. pneumoniae;* and direct fluorescent antibody studies to diagnose *Legionella* species, viruses, and *Pneumocystis carinii.*[4,9]

Traditionally, physicians have drawn simultaneous blood cultures from two different sites. Since the increased sensitivity from drawing two blood cultures seems to be related to the increased volume of blood, rather than the two different sites, it probably does not matter whether the two blood cultures are drawn from the same site or different sites.[2,7] An advantage of using two different sites relates to better information concerning possible skin contaminants.

Consider mycoplasmal pneumonia, Legionnaire's disease, influenza, primary tuberculosis, and other causes of atypical pneumonias in patients with the following clinical findings[1]:

1. Occurrence in young adults

2. Onset over several days

3. Fever not high; patient does not appear severely ill

4. No or small amounts of mucopurulent sputum

5. Minimal pleurisy; small or no effusion

6. Normal to slightly increased white blood cell count

7. Patchy "pneumonitis" or inhomogeneous segmental infiltrate on radiograph

Consider pneumococcal pneumonia, *Haemophilus influenzae*, staphylococcal pneumonia, Gram-negative bacillary pneumonia, and suppurative pulmonary disease in patients with the following clinical findings[1]:

1. Patient more often elderly or chronically ill

2. Abrupt onset

3. High fevers; chills; patient mav appear weak, cyanotic, or confused.

4. Purulent sputum

5. Often has pleurisy and pleural effusion

6. Leukocytosis

7. Lobar or segmental consolidation on radiograph

In debilitated elderly persons and patients with predisposing conditions, probable causative bacteria are as follows[1]:

1. Chronic obstructive pulmonary disease: *S. pneumoniae* and *H. influenzae*.

2. Chronic alcoholism: *S. pneumoniae*, anaerobic bacteria (aspiration pneumonia), *H. influenzae*, *Klebsiella pneumoniae*, *Staphylococcus aureus*, and *Mycobacterium tuberculosis*.

3. Postinfluenza bacterial pneumonia: *S. pneumoniae*, *S. aureus*, and *H. influenzae*.

4. Elderly nursing home patients: *S. pneumoniae*, *S. aureus*, *K. pneumoniae* (and other Gram-negative bacilli), and *H. influenzae*.

5. Patients with mental obtundation, swallowing problems, esophageal disorders, seizure disorders, and poor dental hygiene: usually mixed aerobic/anaerobic bacteria (aspiration pneumonia).

6. Cystic fibrosis: *Pseudomonas aeruginosa* and *S. aureus*.

7. Immunocompromised hosts: multiple etiologies, including Gram-negative bacilli (e.g., *Escherichia coli*, *K. pneumoniae*, *P. aeruginosa*), *S. aureus*, and other bacteria, as well as viral (e.g., cytomegalovirus), fungal (e.g., *Aspergillus*), and protozoal (e.g., *P. carinii*) pathogens. The likely spectrum of causative organisms will vary, depending on the cause of the immunodeficiency (e.g., *S. aureus*, aerobic Gram-negative bacilli, and *Aspergillus* are likely pathogens in neutropenic patients). Although any single test must be interpreted with caution, increasing serum lactate dehydrogenase (LD) levels, particularly over 450 U/L, are suspicious for *P. carinii* in HIV-infected patients with pulmonary disease.[11]

2. In mycoplasmal pneumonia, Legionnaire's disease, influenza, primary tuberculosis, and other causes of atypical pneumonias, laboratory test results are as follows.

MYCOPLASMAL PNEUMONIA

A hemolytic anemia caused by cold agglutinins may occur, but clinically significant hemolysis is rare. A positive direct Coombs' test occurs in up to 83% of patients. The leukocyte count may be normal to slightly increased with a minimal left shift and a possible mild lymphopenia. The erythrocyte sedimentation rate (ESR) increases to over 40 mm/hr in at least two thirds of cases. In the sputum, mononuclear cells predominate over neutrophils in a ratio of about 60/40 (occasionally, neutrophils predominate), and a Gram stain shows no bacteria—there may be some erythrocytes. The organism can be cultured from the sputum or posterior pharynx but takes 2 to 3 weeks to grow. A nucleic acid probe for *Mycoplasma pneumoniae* is available but has not received extensive clinical evaluation. A diagnosis can be made by demonstrating a specific IgM titer of 1:4 or greater or by a single complement-fixing antibody titer of 1:256 or greater. About 50% to 60% of patients show a fourfold or greater rise in the cold agglutinin titer for human type O erythrocytes or a single titer of 1:128 or greater: in sicker patients, cold agglutinins are more likely. Titers of 1:32 or lower can occur in infectious mononucleosis and pneumonia caused by adenovirus or influenza. A cold agglutinin bedside test is available in which 4 or 5 drops of blood are added to a sodium citrate (blue top) vacuum blood collection tube and the tube is immersed in ice water for 30 seconds and then tilted so that blood runs down the side. A positive reaction consists of flocculation that disappears after the tube is incubated at 37°C and correlates well with cold agglutinin titers of 1:64 or greater.[9,V]

LEGIONNAIRE'S DISEASE

The leukocyte count is normal to moderately increased with a left shift. There is moderate neutrophilia in the sputum, and a Gram stain shows weakly staining Gram-negative bacteria. The organism can be cultured from sputum, lung tissue, or pleural fluid and can be directly identified in secretions and tissues using an immunofluorescent technique (for sputum, the sensitivity of the immunofluorescent technique varies from 30% to 70%). Using acute and convalescent sera, 80% of patients have a fourfold rise in titer to 1:128, in 2 to 6 weeks. A single titer of 1:256 or more is also significant. In patients with Legionnaire's disease, an elevated aspartate aminotransferase (AST or SGOT) occurs in 90% of patients.[9]

INFLUENZA

The diagnosis of influenza depends on the clinical findings. Viral culture requires 7 to 10 days. Secondary bacterial pneumonias can be caused by pneumococci, staphylococci, *H. influenzae,* and Gram-negative bacteria, especially *P. aeruginosa.*[8]

PRIMARY TUBERCULOSIS

The diagnosis of primary tuberculosis depends on the clinical findings, radiographs, and results of the tuberculin skin test. Sputum cultures fail to confirm the diagnosis in many adults with mild primary tuberculosis.

OTHER ATYPICAL PNEUMONIAS

Many viral agents, particularly adenoviruses, can mimic mycoplasmal pneumonia. Rare causes include Q fever, psittacosis, tularemia, plague, primary histoplasmosis, and primary coccidioidomycosis.

3. In pneumococcal pneumonia, staphylococcal pneumonia, meningococcal pneumonia, pneumonia caused by *H. influenzae, Branhamella catarrhalis,* and Gram-negative bacilli, laboratory test results are as follows:

Pneumococcal pneumonia accounts for about two thirds of the cases of bacterial pneumonia.[9]

PNEUMOCOCCAL PNEUMONIA

In pneumococcal pneumonia the leukocyte count is usually elevated to 15,000 to 30,000 cells/μL with a left shift and often toxic granulation; however, it may be normal or low. In the sputum, neutrophils are numerous, and the predominant organisms are Gram-positive, lancet-shaped diplococci, which can be cultured. The blood culture is positive in 20% to 30% of patients. If anemia is present, it probably represents a preexisting condition. Hypernatremia caused by loss of free water secondary to fever and sweating may occur.

STAPHYLOCOCCAL PNEUMONIA

In staphylococcal pneumonia the leukocyte count is elevated with a left shift, and the sputum smear shows numerous neutrophils and Gram-positive cocci in clumps, which may be cultured. Blood culture may be positive.

MENINGOCOCCAL PNEUMONIA

In meningococcal pneumonia neutrophilic leukocytosis is usual. The sputum smear shows Gram-negative diplococci that are often present in the cytoplasm of neutrophils. Blood culture may be positive.

PNEUMONIA CAUSED BY *HAEMOPHILUS INFLUENZAE*

In pneumonia caused by *H. influenzae* there is a neutrophilic leukocytosis, and the sputum smear shows abundant pleomorphic Gram-negative organisms, often in neutrophils. About 20% of patients have positive blood cultures.

BRANHAMELLA (NEISSERIA) CATARRHALIS

Formerly regarded as a contaminant, *B. catarrhalis* has emerged as a true pathogen. Patients with chronic obstructive pulmonary disease are susceptible. The bacterium can be recovered from respiratory secretions either in pure culture or occasionally in association with other potentially pathogenic organisms, such as *S. pneumoniae*. Many strains of *B. catarrhalis* are *beta-lactamase* positive.[9]

GRAM-NEGATIVE BACILLARY PNEUMONIAS

In Gram-negative bacillary pneumonias a neutrophilic leukocytosis is typical, but there may be neutropenia. Numerous Gram-negative bacilli are present in the sputum, and these can be cultured. About 20% to 30% of patients have positive blood cultures.

4. In patients with viral, mycoplasmal, or other miscellaneous types of pneumonia, the following additional abnormal laboratory results may occur.

HEMATOLOGY

- Decreased hemoglobin and hematocrit.
- Leukocytosis.
- Although an elevated erythrocyte sedimentation rate (ESR) occurs in mycoplasmal pneumonia, elevated acute-phase reactants are more characteristic of bacterial pneumonia than viral pneumonia; for example, an elevated C-reactive protein (CRP) is said to be useful to distinguish bacterial from viral pneumonia.[6]

CHEMISTRY

- Decreased PO_2 caused by pneumonia
- Abnormal PCO_2 (commonly decreased) caused by pneumonia
- Abnormal total CO_2 caused by change in bicarbonate in compensation for abnormal PCO_2
- Elevated aspartate aminotransferase (AST or SGOT), lactate dehydrogenase (LD), and alkaline phosphate (ALP)

5. In patients with bacterial pneumonia, the following additional abnormal laboratory test results may occur.

HEMATOLOGY

- Decreased hemoglobin and hematocrit
- Leukocytosis, characteristically neutrophilic
- Leukopenia, for example, in fulminating pneumonococcal pneumonia in alcoholics
- Elevated ESR and acute-phase reactant (CRP)

CHEMISTRY

- Decreased PO_2 caused by pneumonia
- Abnormal PCO_2 (commonly decreased) caused by pneumonia
- Abnormal total CO_2 caused by change in bicarbonate in compensation for abnormal PCO_2
- Elevated aspartate aminotransferase (AST or SGOT) and lactate dehydrogenase (LD)
- Decreased albumin
- Elevated bilirubin

REFERENCES

1. American Medical Association Department of Drugs, Division of Drugs and Technology: Drug Evaluations, 6th ed. Chicago, American Medical Association, 1986, p 1238.
2. Gambino R: Blood cultures: Two-site vs one-site. Lab Report for Physicians 9:93, 1987.

3. Harris GD, Johanson WG: Cough, fever, chill (pneumococcal pneumonia). In Cutler P: Problem Solving in Clinical Medicine: From Data to Diagnosis, 2nd ed. Baltimore, Williams & Wilkins, 1985, p 344.
4. Kovacs JA, Ng VL, Masur H, et al: Diagnosis of *Pneumocystis carinii* pneumonia: Improved detection in sputum with use of monoclonal antibodies. N Engl J Med 318:589, 1988.
5. Lentino JR, Lucks DA: Nonvalue of sputum culture in the management of lower respiratory tract infections. J Clin Microbiol 25:758, 1987.
6. McCarthy PL, Frank AL, Ablow RC, et al: Value of C-reactive protein in differentiation of bacterial and viral pneumonia. J Pediatr 92:454, 1978.
7. Plorde JJ, Tenover FC, Carlson LG: Specimen volume versus yield in the BACTEC blood culture system. J Clin Microbiol 22:292, 1985.
8. Proceedings of a Symposium. Prevention, management, and control of influenza: A mandate for the 1980's. Am J Med 82(6A), 1987.
9. Pulmonary Medicine Subspecialty Committee: Medical Knowledge Self-Assessment Program VIII. Pulmonary Medicine. Philadelphia, American College of Physicians, 1988, p 237.
10. Sears DA: Cough, fever, then fatigue (pneumococcal pneumonia). In Cutler P: Problem Solving in Clinical Medicine: From Data to Diagnosis, 2nd ed. Baltimore, Williams & Wilkins, 1985, p 245.
11. Zaman M, White DA: Serum lactate dehydrogenase levels and *Pneumocystis carinii* pneumonia. Am Rev Respir Dis 137:796, 1988.

PLEURAL EFFUSION

Normally, pleural fluid is absorbed by the visceral pleura as it is produced by the parietal pleura, so that only a minimal amount of free fluid is present in the pleural spaces of healthy individuals. Five pathophysiologic mechanisms can cause abnormally large amounts of pleural fluid to accumulate (a pleural effusion): (1) increased hydrostatic pressure, as in congestive heart failure; (2) increased capillary permeability, as in pneumonia or any type of pleurisy; (3) decreased oncotic pressure, as in hypoalbuminemia; (4) increased intrapleural negative pressure, as in atelectasis; and (5) impaired lymphatic drainage of the pleural space, as in mediastinal carcinomatosis. A pleural effusion can be discovered by clinical findings and radiographic studies. The evaluation of a pleural effusion centers on distinguishing transudative effusions from exudative effusions. Transudates are commonly caused by congestive heart failure and low-protein states, and, once identified, do not require further laboratory investigation. On the other hand, exudates are caused by neoplasms, infections, and other inflammations and require additional laboratory studies to diagnose the specific neoplasm or infection or to further categorize the inflammation.[2,4]

1. In patients with a pleural effusion, to diagnose the cause of the effusion, perform a thoracentesis and request pleural fluid total protein and lactate dehydrogenase (LD), together with serum total protein and LD. A pleural fluid cholesterol may be helpful.

The appearance of the pleural fluid can offer clues concerning its etiology. For example, transudates are usually clear and straw colored, whereas exudates can be turbid, purulent, or bloody. It takes about 10,000 erythrocytes per cubic millimeter to impart a pink color to the fluid. A milky appearance suggests a chylous effusion. Light[5] established the validity of using pleural and serum protein and LD measurements to distinguish pleural fluid exudates from transudates.

Collect pleural fluid for appropriate tests and one tube of venous blood as follows: (1) pleural fluid for chemistry tests: 10 ml, heparinized (glucose can decrease if the fluid is not frozen or preserved with fluoride); (2) venous blood for chemistry tests: one clot tube (glucose can decrease if the serum is not frozen or preserved with fluoride); (3) pleural fluid for cytology: 25 to 50 ml, heparinized; (4) pleural fluid for bacterial cultures: 10 ml, heparinized; (5) pleural fluid for acid-fast and fungal cultures: 10 ml, heparinized; (5) pleural fluid for acid-fast and fungal cultures: 10 ml, heparinized (a larger quantity, i.e., 50 ml, increases the sensitivity for culturing acid-fast bacilli); (6) pleural fluid for hematology tests: one EDTA tube; (7) pleural fluid for pH: several milliliters collected anaerobically, iced, and quickly sent to the laboratory; and (8) pleural fluid for miscellaneous tests: 10 ml, heparinized. These samples should be delivered to the laboratory immediately.[1]

2. Evaluate the tests.

SENSITIVITY AND SPECIFICITY OF TESTS USED FOR CLASSIFICATION OF PLEURAL EFFUSION

TEST	EXUDATE	SENSITIVITY (%)	SPECIFICITY (%)
1. Specific gravity	>1.016	78	89
2. Pleural fluid protein	>3 g	93	85
3. Pleural fluid/serum protein	>0.5	92	93
4. Pleural fluid LD*	>200	72	100
5. Pleural fluid/serum LD	>0.6	88	96
Test 3 or 5 positive	—	99	89
Tests 3 and 5 positive	—	81	100

Source: Reprinted with permission from Skendzel LP: A practical approach to the chemical and microscopic study of pleural and peritoneal fluids. Labmedica V(1):15, 1988.

*LD method with a reference range of <300 U/L. Current LD methods may not be comparable.

The leukocyte count is usually less than 1000/mm^3 in transudates. More than 80% of transudates but less than 20% of exudates have leukocyte counts below 1000/mm^3.

Of 62 effusions studied, a pleural fluid cholesterol level above 60 mg/dl (1.6 mmol/L) correctly identified all but three pleural exudates. Transudates had lower levels.[3]

3. If the pleural fluid/serum protein and pleural fluid/serum LD indicate that the fluid is a transudate, no further testing is usually necessary.

A recent study of 533 pleural fluid specimens from 340 patients showed that an average of 8.7 tests were performed on each fluid, including WBC, WBC differential, and other specific studies. Although these may prove useful when the fluid is an exudate, they are of little use when the fluid is a transudate and further testing is not required.[6]

4. If the pleural fluid/serum protein and/or pleural fluid/serum LD studies indicate that the fluid is an exudate, the following tests may prove useful: pH; glucose; amylase; rheumatoid factor, antinuclear antibodies (ANAs), lupus erythematosus (LE) cells and complement; erythrocyte count; triglycerides; biopsy; cytology; and cultures for bacteria, acid-fast, and fungal organisms.

USEFUL TESTS IN PLEURAL FLUID EXUDATES

TEST	DISEASES
pH (<7.20)	Infection, malignancy, rheumatoid arthritis, esophageal rupture
Glucose (<60 mg/dl [3.33 mmol/L])	Infection, malignancy, rheumatoid arthritis
Amylase (>200 U/L)	Pancreatic disease, malignancy, esophageal rupture
Rheumatoid factor, ANA, LE cells, complement (decreased)	Collagen vascular disease, lupus erythematosus, rheumatoid arthritis
Cytology, biopsy	Malignancy, tuberculosis
Erythrocytes (>100,000/μl)	Pulmonary embolus, malignancy, trauma
Chylous effusion (triglycerides >100 mg/dl [1.14 mmol/L])	Trauma, malignancy

In lieu of a biopsy, which requires a physician experienced in the technique, cytologic studies using Wright-Giemsa– and Pap-stained preparations by an experienced laboratory can be extremely useful in identifying the cause of an effusion. Cytologic study has a higher diagnostic yield than pleural biopsy in malignant disease of the pleura but a lower yield than pleural biopsy for tuberculous disease of the pleura. A leukocyte differential count that shows over 50% lymphocytes suggests tuberculosis or neoplasm; a count of greater than 50% polymorphonuclear cells suggests acute inflammation. Grossly bloody fluid may be seen with pulmonary infarction, tumor, or trauma.[7,VI]

REFERENCES

1. Gambino R (ed): Pleural effusion. Lab Report for Physicians 2:75, 1980.
2. Hall WJ: Pleural effusions. In Griner PF, Panzer RJ, Greenland P: Clinical Diagnosis and the Laboratory: Logical Strategies for Common Medical Problems. Chicago, Year Book Medical Publishers, Inc, 1986, p 183.
3. Hamm H, Brohan U, Bohmer R, et al: Cholesterol in pleural effusions: A diagnostic aid. Chest 92:296, 1987.
4. Harris GD, Johanson WG: Sudden shortness of breath (pleural effusion). In Cutler P: Problem Solving in Clinical Medicine: From Data to Diagnosis, 2nd ed. Baltimore, Williams & Wilkins, 1985, p 349.
5. Light RW: Pleural Diseases. Philadelphia, Lea & Febiger, 1983.
6. Peterman TA, Speicher CE: Evaluating pleural effusions: A two-stage laboratory approach. JAMA 252:1051, 1984.
7. Skendzel LP: A practical approach to the chemical and microscopic study of pleural and peritoneal fluids. Labmedica V(1):15, 1988.

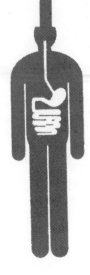

CHAPTER 5

ACUTE DIARRHEA

INTESTINAL MALABSORPTION

ASCITES

GASTROINTESTINAL DISORDERS

ACUTE DIARRHEA

Acute diarrhea is diarrhea of less than a week's duration that is characterized by an increase in daily stool weight of more than 250 g, liquidity, and a frequency of more than three bowel movements per day. It is usually self-limited and requires no treatment; however, it may be prolonged and reflect serious disease, that is, dysentery. Dysentery refers to severe inflammation of the intestine, usually the colon, associated with blood, pus, and mucus in the stool. In third world countries, it is estimated that there are 3 to 5 billion episodes of acute diarrhea annually, with 5 to 10 million deaths. In the United States, diarrheal diseases are also common but are less morbid. Recently, the high annual death rate in the United States among children (100) and infants (400) has been emphasized.[4] The etiologies include viruses, bacteria, bacterial toxins, parasites, diarrhea associated with systemic infections, and miscellaneous causes. In the strategy that follows, a key tactic is to differentiate noninflammatory diarrhea from inflammatory diarrhea using the number of polymorphonuclear leukocytes in the fecal smear. This test, when taken together with the clinical findings, does a reasonably good job of separating the two types of diarrhea. Notable exceptions are mentioned throughout the discussion.[1-3,5,8,10]

1.   In patients with acute diarrhea that persists for more than several days in whom toxicity and fecal blood are absent, examine a fecal smear for polymorphonuclear leukocytes to distinguish the clinical syndromes of noninflammatory diarrhea from the inflammatory types of diarrhea. Occult blood testing may also be helpful.

Apply a thin layer of feces or mucus to a slide, mix with one drop of Loeffler's methylene blue, seal with a coverslip, and examine for polymorphonuclear leukocytes (Wright's stain may also be used). More than five leukocytes per high-power field in five or more fields is considered positive for inflammatory diarrhea. Erythrocytes or occult blood suggests an inflammatory cause, but there are exceptions, such as ischemia.[10]

Acute diarrhea may be divided into two types, noninflammatory and inflammatory, on the basis of whether or not there are polymorphonuclear leukocytes in the feces. This is a clinically relevant classification, since in the United States, noninflammatory disease tends to be self-limited and is associated with cramping, bloating, periumbilical pain, and large-volume, watery stools. Fever, leukocytosis, and constitutional symptoms are absent. In contrast, inflammatory diarrhea or dysentery is associated with mucosal invasion and commonly accompanied by fever, other constitutional symptoms, lower abdominal pain, and tenesmus. Stools may be small in volume and often are bloody or mucoid.[10]

69

2. If the fecal smear shows five or fewer polymorphonuclear leukocytes per high-power field, the diarrhea is probably noninflammatory and the illness will usually be self-limited.

In the United States Norwalk virus and other viral agents are the most common causes of noninflammatory diarrhea in adults. The diarrhea is explosive and lasts about 24 to 48 hours. Rotavirus infection predominates in infants and young children and produces severely watery diarrhea of 5 to 8 days' duration. Other causes of noninflammatory diarrhea include enterotoxigenic *Escherichia coli*, *Vibrio cholerae*, and *Giardia lamblia*, as well as bacterial toxins associated with food poisoning (*Staphylococcus* and *Clostridium perfringens*). These organisms or toxins do not invade the mucosa but induce a secretory, watery diarrhea; thus fecal leukocytes are typically absent.[10]

Remember that some inflammatory diarrheas will not show more than five polymorphonuclear leukocytes per high-power field. These inflammatory diarrheas can thus appear to be noninflammatory diarrhea. For example, this may happen with approximately 30% of *Shigella* infections, and similar results have been reported for *Campylobacter* infections. In antibiotic-associated colitis (especially clindamycin, lincomycin, ampicillin, and cephalosporins), leukocytes are few or absent when the process is limited but are common in diffuse disease. Likewise, *Entamoeba histolytica*, *Salmonella*, *Yersinia enterocolitica*, and *Vibrio parahaemolyticus* infections produce variable findings, and the presence of leukocytes depends on the degree of colonic invasion.[10]

There are a number of noninfectious causes of noninflammatory diarrhea. Drugs that can cause diarrhea include laxatives, warfarin, thyroid hormones, magnesium-containing antacids, quinidine, colchicine, cholestyramine, digoxin, and antimetabolites. Diarrhea can occur with toxins such as heavy metals (lead, zinc, cadmium, copper), poisonous fish (ciguatoxin, scombrotoxin, puffer fish, shellfish), monosodium glutamate, botulism, and mushroom poisoning. Fecal impaction is an additional cause. Some patients with irritable bowel or an inflamed rectum may pass several loose bowel movements each day that do not exceed 250g. Diabetic diarrhea is common in patients with diabetic peripheral and autonomic neuropathy, and bacterial overgrowth may play a role.[2,V]

When the cause of diarrhea is noninflammatory and noninfectious, for diagnostic purposes, it may be useful to distinguish osmotic diarrhea from secretory diarrhea. Osmotic diarrhea is caused by the accumulation of nonabsorbable solutes in the gut lumen, such as divalent or trivalent ions (Mg^{++}, $PO_4^=$, $SO_4^=$) in saline laxatives and lactose secondary to disaccharidase deficiency. In contrast, secretory diarrhea (usually over 1000 ml/day) is caused by a net luminal gain of secretions, that is, electrolytes and water. Examples of secretory diarrhea include enterotoxin-induced diarrhea, pancreatic cholera syndrome, carcinoid syndrome, glucagonoma, Zollinger-Ellison syndrome (tumor can be demonstrated by CT scan or peptide assay), and surreptitious ingestion of cathartic agents such as phenolphthalein (pink color of alkalinized stool). Osmotic diarrhea can be distinguished from secretory diarrhea by calculating the stool osmolal gap as follows: Stool osmolal gap = Measured stool osmolality − $2[(Na^+) + (K^+)]$. If the stool osmolal gap is positive (high), it indicates an osmotic diarrhea. If it is negative, it indicates a secretory diarrhea. The stool sample must be fresh or stored at 4°C. Measured osmolality of diarrheal stool is 285 to

330 mOsm/kg, and in osmotic diarrhea, the stool osmolal gap is typically over 160 mOsm/kg (alternatively, in secretory diarrhea, the fecal $Na^+ + K^+$ are about equal to one half of the serum osmolality). Osmotic diarrhea typically stops after a 24-hour fast, whereas secretory diarrhea persists.[2,6]

Watery diarrhea can also occur with other chronic conditions: irritable bowel syndrome, inflammatory bowel disease, villous adenoma, ischemic colitis, and mesenteric thrombosis.

3.   If the fecal smear shows greater than five polymorphonuclear leukocytes per high-power field, the diarrhea is probably inflammatory and the cause should be determined. The presence of erythrocytes or occult blood suggests an inflammatory cause.

Polymorphonuclear leukocytes are specific for colonic inflammation and suggest infection from *Shigella, Salmonella, Yersinia, Campylobacter,* invasive *Escherichia coli, Giardia,* antibiotic-associated colitis, ulcerative colitis, and ischemic colitis. During the summer months or if seafood has been eaten, consider *V. parahaemolyticus.* Fecal occult blood testing is not as useful as examination for leukocytes, but when combined with leukocytes it can increase the positive predictive value for bacterial infection.[7] Chronic inflammatory disease of the colon (ulcerative colitis and Crohn's disease) yields low-volume diarrhea (<1000 ml/day) containing many leukocytes.[2,6,10]

4.   Perform stool cultures and stool examination for ova and parasites in the following situations: fecal blood (gross or occult), fecal leukocytes, temperature above 38.3°C (101°F), admission to the hospital, food handlers, persistent diarrhea, diarrhea associated with debilitation, travelers with a history of exposure, and epidemiologic considerations. Avoid barium enema examination.

If *Campylobacter jejuni* or *V. parahaemolyticus* is suspected, request selective culture techniques. Request gonorrheal identification in homosexual men, and remember that homosexual men are at increased risks for infections with *Salmonella, Shigella, Campylobacter, G. lamblia, E. histolytica, Chlamydia trachomatis,* and Herpes simplex. Consider parasites with these findings: undiagnosed diarrhea for longer than 1 week, travel history of exposure, and homosexual exposure to amebiasis or giardiasis. Three different stool specimens promptly delivered to the laboratory are best for diagnosis. Avoid barium enema examination, enemas, laxatives, and antibiotics, since these can obscure the diagnosis. In patients in whom clinical suspicion of parasitism persists and all three stool examinations are negative, additional specimens should be examined.[9] Patients with acquired immunodeficiency syndrome (AIDS) are susceptible to infections with *Cryptosporidium,* cytomegalovirus, herpes simplex virus, *Candida albicans,* and *Mycobacterium avium-intracellulare.*[2,10]

5.   Perform proctosigmoidoscopy in patients with toxicity, bloody diarrhea, antibiotic-associated diarrhea, or prolonged diarrhea.

Sigmoidoscopy will reveal the yellow-gray plaques of antibiotic-associated colitis, and the diagnosis can be confirmed by rectal biopsy, measuring *Clostrid-*

ium difficile toxin, or anaerobic culture of *C. difficile.* In amebiasis there will be colonic ulcerations containing amoebas, and serologic tests using gel diffusion precipitin or indirect hemagglutination tests are positive in 85% to 95% of patients. In ulcerative colitis, the rectal and colonic mucosa will be diffusely red and friable, and cultures will be negative. Consider ischemic colitis with these findings: older patients with atherosclerotic vascular disease and with diarrhea. A barium enema examination may be useful to diagnosis ischemic colitis ever though it is ordinarily not part of the evaluation of acute diarrhea.[10]

6.   In patients with acute diarrhea, the following additional abnormal laboratory test results may occur:

HEMATOLOGY

- Elevated hemoglobin and hematocrit caused by loss of salt and water with contraction of the extracellular compartment and hemoconcentration
- Leukocytosis with inflammatory diarrhea

CHEMISTRY

- Metabolic acidosis
- Elevated urea and creatinine associated with prerenal azotemia
- Hypernatremia and elevated chloride with dehydration related to water loss (With diarrhea, hypokalemia and decreased carbon dioxide may occur. If water is replaced and not electrolytes, decreased sodium, potassium, chloride, carbon dioxide, and urea may occur.)
- Elevated albumin and calcium (bound to albumin) with dehydration
- Elevated alkaline phosphatase (intestinal type) in ulcerative lesions of the intestine, such as ulcerative colitis

REFERENCES

1. Bruckstein AH: Acute diarrhea. AFP 38:217, 1988.
2. Gastroenterology Subspecialty Committee: Medical Knowledge Self-Assessment Program VIII. Gastroenterology. Philadelphia, American College of Physicians, 1988, p 419.
3. Ho M, Glass RI, Pinsky PF, et al: Diarrheal deaths in American children. Are they preventable? JAMA 260:3281, 1988.
4. Levine JS: Decision Making in Gastroenterology. St Louis, The CV Mosby Co, 1985, p 66.
5. Satterwhite TK, DuPont HL: Acute diarrhea. In Lundberg GD (ed): Using the Clinical Laboratory in Medical Decision-Making. Chicago, American Society of Clinical Pathologists, 1983, p 55.
6. Shiau Y, Feldman GM, Resnick MA, et al: Stool electrolyte and osmolality measurements in the evaluation of diarrheal disorders. Ann Intern Med 102:773, 1985.
7. Siegel D, Cohen PT, Neighbor M, et al: Predictive value of stool examination in acute diarrhea. Arch Pathol Lab Med 111:715, 1987.
8. Suchman AL, Griner PF: Acute diarrhea. In Griner PF, Panzer RJ, Greenland P: Clinical Diagnosis and the Laboratory: Logical Strategies for Common Medical Problems. Chicago, Year Book Publishers, Inc, 1986, p 333.
9. Thomson RB, Haas RA: Intestinal parasites: The necessity of examining multiple stool specimens. Mayo Clin Proc 59:641, 1984.
10. Tolle SW, Elliot DL: The evaluation and management of acute diarrhea. West J Med 140:293, 1984.

INTESTINAL MALABSORPTION

Steatorrhea, or intestinal malabsorption, is a type of chronic diarrhea that must be distinguished from other causes of chronic diarrhea, such as irritable bowel and inflammatory bowel disease. Malabsorption is a term used to indicate defective absorption of nutrients by the small intestine. These nutrients include fats, proteins, carbohydrates, vitamins, and minerals, individually or in combination. The defective absorption may be caused by intestinal, biliary, or pancreatic disease. In biliary or pancreatic disease, the intestine may be normal and the disorder is more appropriately called maldigestion. When the defective absorption is caused by intestinal disease, the disorder is sometimes referred to as malassimilation. The diagnosis and management of intestinal malabsorption are by a combination of clinical findings, radiographic studies, and laboratory tests. Laboratory tests are used to determine whether malabsorption exists and, if it does, whether it is caused by disorders of the intestine, pancreas, or biliary tract. A key clinical feature is the marked difficulty the patient describes in flushing stool down the toilet because of increased stool volume and fat content (when fecal fat is about 20 g/day, at least two flushings are required to clear the toilet water). Common symptoms include weight loss, abdominal distention, pain, diarrhea, and flatulence.[3,5,7,8,V]

1. In patients with clinical findings of steatorrhea, obtain a 72-hour stool collection for quantitative fecal fat analysis. To perform a 72-hour fecal fat analysis place the individual to be tested on an 80 to 100 g/day fat diet* and continue this diet during the collection period. Microscopic examination of a random stool sample may be used as a qualitative screening test. Serum carotene and vitamin A levels may be helpful.

Although microscopic examination of a random stool sample may be used as a screening test, quantitative documentation of increased fecal fat over a 3-day period is the best method for diagnosing intestinal malabsorption. Serum carotene and vitamin A levels may be depressed, but these tests are not reliable enough to use as diagnostic tests.

2. To perform a microscopic examination for increased fecal fat obtain a random stool sample and proceed in the following manner.[2,6]

When done properly, the Sudan stain has an 80% to 90% sensitivity for detecting clinically significant steatorrhea.[7]

1. Place a small amount of stool (size of one half of a split pea) on a glass slide. If not liquid, add several drops of water or saline and make a homogenate by using applicator stick as a pestle.

---

*The patient should not ingest castor, mineral, or nut oils and should not use suppositories. After 3 to 5 days of the diet, begin a 72-hour stool collection for quantitative fecal fat analysis. Collect the specimens in glass or plastic containers (clean paint cans work well). Wax-coated containers should not be used. During the collection period, the fecal specimens should be refrigerated, and contamination of feces with urine should be avoided. Any obvious foreign matter should be removed before proceeding with the analysis.

2. Add 2 or 3 drops of glacial acetic acid and 4 or 5 drops of alcoholic solution of Sudan stain, mix, and add coverslip.

3. Heat with alcohol lamp or burner to boiling to facilitate hydrolysis of soaps to free fatty acids and to facilitate staining.

4. Examine under a microscope while slide is warm using low power to locate stained fat droplets and high power to examine droplets.

> NORMAL: A few small droplets should be noticeable and represent normal fat excretion; these reassure the examiner that the slide has been prepared properly.

> ABNORMAL: A much larger number and size of reddish-colored round droplets indicate steatorrhea.

5. Pitfalls: The skillful examiner gains experience by comparing examination of stool from patients with steatorrhea with that from normal individuals. False-positive results may occur in patients receiving castor oil, mineral oil, and oil-based suppositories. False-negative results may result from barium diluting the stool. Failure to examine the slide while warm may result in conversion of the stained melted fat droplets to unstained needlelike crystals. If this occurs, the slide should be reheated and reexamined.

3. Evaluate the tests.

REFERENCE RANGE VALUES[6,x]

TEST	SPECIMEN	REFERENCE RANGE (CONVENTIONAL)	REFERENCE RANGE (INTERNATIONAL)
Fat, fecal	Feces (72 hr)	<7 g/day	<7 g/day
Beta-carotene	Serum	60–200 μg/dl	1.12–3.72 μmol/L
Vitamin A	Serum	30–65 μg/dl	1.05–2.27 μmol/L

TEST	NORMAL FAT EXCRETERS (<6 g/24 hr)	ABNORMAL FAT EXCRETERS (>6 g/24 hr)
Number of microscopic fat droplets[6] per high-lower field	2.5 ± 0.8	26.6 ± 4.0

The ^{14}C-triolein breath test is another screening test for steatorrhea. Compared with the quantitative fecal fat test, it has a sensitivity of 85% to 100% and a specificity of 93% to 96%. False-positive results with the breath test can occur in patients with obesity, gastric retention, and chronic liver disease.[7,v]

4. If fecal fat is elevated, the patient has malabsorption. Perform a xylose absorption test to differentiate maldigestion (pancreatic disease) from malassimilation (intestinal disease). A small bowel series is appropriate.

The degree of fecal fat elevation is not useful in differentiating between pancreatic and intestinal disease.[4] To perform the xylose absorption test the patient ingests 25 g of xylose and collects urine for the next 5 hours. It is important that the patient drink 500 ml of water during the first 3 hours of the collection period to ensure adequate urinary filtration of the xylose. A normal xylose absorption test shows 10 to 20 mg/dl/1.73 m^2 (0.67 to 1.33 mmol/L/1.73m^2) of body surface area elevation of the serum level within 60 to 75 minutes after ingestion of xylose, or 5 g or more of xylose in the urine within 5 hours. False-positive xylose absorption tests occasionally occur in the following situations:[7,V]

1. Decreased renal function in patients over 60 years of age or patient of any age with renal disease (false-positive urine test but serum test is valid)

2. Patients with increased extracellular fluid, particularly with ascites or massive edema

3. Patients with delayed gastric emptying (can be overcome by instilling the test dose through a tube directly into the proximal intestine)

In patients with decreased renal function, only serum levels should be used in the interpretation of xylose absorption.

A small bowel series can suggest the presence of malabsorption and help differentiate intraluminal maldigestion from malassimilation.[7]

5.   If fecal fat is elevated and the xylose absorption test is abnormal, consider intestinal disease.

In this circumstance, a small bowel biopsy can be useful to diagnose such intestinal diseases as celiac sprue, Whipple's disease, hypogammaglobulinemia (IgA), lymphangiectasia, and lymphoma. A recent study suggests that the xylose absorption test is not useful to diagnose adult celiac disease or to monitor the effect of dietary treatment.[1] A normal biopsy result suggests bacterial overgrowth (10^5 organisms per milliliter of jejunal fluid on quantitative culture or an elevated ^{14}C-xylose or ^{14}C-glycocholate breath test). The most common disorders of the small bowel that lead to malabsorption (other than bowel resection) are celiac disease, tropical sprue, and bacterial overgrowth.[3]

6.   If fecal fat is elevated and the xylose absorption test is normal, consider biliary or pancreatic disease. Evaluate the patient for diabetes mellitus and perform appropriate radiographic and endoscopic studies.

Pancreatic diabetes occurs in one third of all patients with chronic pancreatitis and in approximately twice this number of patients with calcific pancreatitis. Radiographic and sometimes endoscopic studies are necessary to adequately evaluate the patient. Although the secretin, cholecystokinin stimulation, and Lundh tests are useful, they are not commonly performed, because they require intubation, which is time consuming and cumbersome. The bentiromide assay is a noninvasive test (85% to 97% sensitive) for detecting advanced chronic pancreatitis or cancer of the pancreatic head with ductal obstruction. When 500 mg of bentiromide is ingested, patients with normal amounts of trypsin excrete at least 50% of the bentiromide as aminobenzoic acid (PABA) in the urine within 6 hours. Patients with pancreatic disease excrete less. Fasting serum trypsinogen is another test to detect chronic pancreatitis or cancer of the pancreatic head causing ductal obstruction. Normally, it is 25 to 80 ng/ml, but in patients with these disorders, it is 2 to 19 ng/ml. Also, other decreased serum analytes can detect chronic pancreatitis, such as pancreatic isoamylase, lipase, and pancreatic polypeptide. Unfortunately, the noninvasive tests of pancreatic function tend to be positive only in severe pancreatic insufficiency, but not in milder forms of the disease.[3,7,V]

7. If the fecal fat excretion is normal, intestinal malabsorption is ruled out, but remember that fecal fat excretion may be normal in specific absorption defects, such as disaccharidase deficiency.

Disaccharidase deficiency, which can be caused by giardiasis, can be diagnosed by an assay of tissue from the small intestine by peroral biopsy. Usually this is not necessary, because the clinical findings can be produced by ingestion of 50 g of the sugar and because dramatic improvement results when milk products are eliminated from the diet. In the oral lactose tolerance test in a fasting patient, a normal individual will show a 20 to 30 mg/dl (1.11 to 1.67 mmol/L) increase in serum glucose in the first 2 hours after ingesting 50 g of lactose. A lactose breath test is also available.[7]

8. In patients with intestinal malabsorption, the following additional abnormal laboratory test results may occur:

HEMATOLOGY

- Elevated hematocrit suggests dehydration.
- Depressed hematocrit suggests blood loss or anemia caused by malabsorption, for example, iron, folate, vitamin B_{12}.*
- Lymphopenia may indicate excessive leakage of lymph into the gut.
- Eosinophilia suggests parasites or eosinophilic gastroenteritis.
- Thrombocytosis suggests ulcerative colitis, Whipple's disease, and celiac sprue.
- Elevated prothrombin time may be caused by impaired absorption of vitamin K.*

CHEMISTRY

- Chronic diarrhea can cause metabolic acidosis or metabolic alkalosis with decreased or increased CO_2 with reciprocal changes in chloride.
- Elevated glucose from pancreatic diabetes.
- Decreased glucose and urea nitrogen may be caused by malabsorption of glucose and protein.
- Elevated sodium and urea nitrogen suggest dehydration.
- Hypokalemia and hyponatremia may be caused by diarrhea.
- Hypocalcemia related to either hypoalbuminemia and/or vitamin D deficiency with decreased calcium absorption. Rare in pancreatic insufficiency.*

---

*Since the absorption of carotene, vitamin K, vitamin D, folate, and iron is independent of pancreatic enzyme digestion, the presence of a low serum carotene, hypocalcemia, hypoprothrombinemia, or anemia suggests a small bowel disorder rather than a pancreatic disorder.

- Hypomagnesemia; rare in pancreatic insufficiency.
- Elevated lactate dehydrogenase (LD) and aspartate aminotransferase (AST or SGOT) from decreased vitamin B_{12} absorption with megaloblastic anemia and intramedullary death of megaloblasts.
- Elevated alkaline phosphatase caused by vitamin D deficiency with decreased calcium absorption causing osteomalacia.
- Hypoalbuminemia.
- Decreased bilirubin related to hypoalbuminemia.
- Hypocholesterolemia.

REFERENCES

1. Bode S, Gudmand-Hoyer E: The diagnostic value of the D-xylose absorption test in adult coeliac disease. Scand J Gasteroenterol 22:1217, 1987.
2. Gambino R: Fecal fat. Lab Report for Physicians 3:57, 1981.
3. Gastroenterology Subspecialty Committee. Medical Knowledge Self-Assessment Program VIII. Gastroenterology. Philadelphia, American College of Physicians, 1988, pp 419, 426.
4. Lembicke B, Grimm K, Lankisch PG: Raised fecal fat concentration is not a valid indicator of pancreatic steatorrhea. Am J Gastroenterol 82:526, 1987.
5. Levine JS: Decision Making in Gastroenterology. St Louis, The CV Mosby Co, 1985, p 98.
6. Simko V: Fecal fat microscopy. Acceptable predictive value in screening for steatorrhea. Am J Gastroenterol 75:204, 1981.
7. Trier JS: Intestinal malabsorption: Differentiation of cause. Hosp Pract 23:195, 1988.
8. Weser E: Diarrhea and weight loss (steatorrhea). In Cutler P: Problem Solving in Clinical Medicine: From Data to Diagnosis, 2nd ed. Baltimore, Williams & Wilkins, 1985, p 382.

ASCITES

Ascites is the accumulation of excessive fluid in the peritoneal cavity. Portal hypertension may be present. The cause of ascites with portal hypertension is almost always cirrhosis or cardiac disease (right ventricular failure or constrictive pericarditis). The causes of ascites without portal hypertension are many, for example, cancer, tuberculosis. Recently, a new strategy for evaluating patients with ascites has been described that is based on the gradient of albumin concentration between serum and ascitic fluid. A high gradient indicates the presence of portal hypertension, and a low gradient indicates its absence. Recently, the term "portal hypertensive ascites" has been used for transudative ascites and "nonportal hypertensive ascites" for exudative ascites.[1-5]

1. In patients with ascites, to diagnose the cause of the ascites, perform a paracentesis and measure ascitic-fluid albumin, total protein, lactate dehydrogenase (LD), and leukocyte count (WBC) together with serum albumin, total protein, and LD.

The gradient (difference) between the serum albumin and ascitic-fluid albumin accurately reflects the oncotic pressure of ascitic fluid and has real pathophysiologic significance. It provides a new way to categorize patients with ascites.

2. Evaluate the tests.

REFERENCE RANGE VALUES: GRADIENT OF SERUM ALBUMIN MINUS ASCITIC-FLUID ALBUMIN (ALBS-A)[3,4]

ASCITES	REFERENCE RANGE (CONVENTIONAL)	REFERENCE RANGE (INTERNATIONAL)
With portal hypertension	≥ 1.1 g/dl	≥ 11 g/L
Without portal hypertension	<1.1 g/dl	<11 g/L

SENSITIVITY AND SPECIFICITY OF TESTS FOR DIFFERENTIATING BETWEEN TRANSUDATIVE AND EXUDATIVE ASCITIC EFFUSIONS

TEST	EXUDATE CRITERIA	SENSITIVITY (%)	SPECIFICITY (%)
Total protein	>3 g/dl (30 g/L)	86	83
Ascitic fluid/serum protein ratio	>0.5	93	85
Ascitic fluid/serum LD ratio	>0.6	79	92
LD	>400 Sigma units (SU)*	57	100
WBC	$>500/mm^3$	—	90
2, 3, and 4 positive		57	100
Serum albumin minus ascitic-fluid albumin	≥ 1.1 g/dl (11 g/L)	87	78

Source: Reprinted with permission from Skendzel LP: A practical approach to the chemical and microscopic study of pleural and peritoneal fluids. Labmedica V(1):15, 1988.
*Normal serum range, 200–500 Sigma units.

3. If the Albs-a is equal to or greater than 1.1 g/dl (11 g/L), conclude that portal hypertension (transudative ascites) is present, which is consistent with cirrhosis or cardiac disease.

There are occasional exceptions when the Albs-a is 1.1 g/dl or greater without portal vein hypertension, notably extensive liver metastases or portal vein thrombosis. An Albs-a gradient of 1.1 g/dl or greater is maintained in patients with cirrhosis, even when a complicating process such as peritoneal tuberculosis develops. The presence of positive exudate criteria, such as an elevated ascitic-fluid WBC, in a patient with portal hypertension and an Albs-a gradient of 1.1 g/dl or greater suggests a second process, such as peritoneal tuberculosis.

4. If the Albs-a gradient is below 1.1 g/dl (11 g/L), conclude that portal hypertension is absent (exudative ascites) and consider other causes for ascites.

Rarely, portal hypertension may be minimal enough in patients with cirrhosis to produce an Albs-a gradient below 1.1 g/dl. In most instances, a low gradient suggests causes not associated with portal hypertension, such as leaking ducts (thoracic, pancreatic, biliary), peritoneal implants (cancer or tuberculosis), myxedema, systemic lupus erythematosus, certain benign ovarian diseases, and severe hypoalbuminemia. Positive exudate criteria are characteristic of a number of the above disorders.

Useful diagnostic studies for ascites without portal hypertension (exudative ascites) include cytology and cultures. A high-protein, exudative ascites with negative cytology suggests infection such as tuberculosis or fungal disease.

REFERENCES

1. Bentch HL: Swelling of the abdomen (ascites). In Cutler P: Problem Solving in Clinical Medicine: From Data to Diagnosis. Baltimore, Williams & Wilkins, 1985, p 527.
2. Levine JS: Decision Making in Gastroenterology. St Louis, The CV Mosby Co, 1985, p 84.
3. Mauer K, Manzione NC: Usefulness of serum-ascites albumin difference in separating transudative from exudative ascites. Another look. Digestive Dis Sci 33:1208, 1988.
4. Rector WG: An improved diagnostic approach to ascites. Arch Intern Med 147:215, 1987.
5. Skendzel LP: A practical approach to the chemical and microscopic study of pleural and peritoneal fluids. Labmedica V(1):15, 1988.

CHAPTER 6

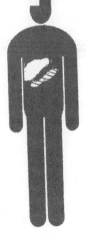

DISORDERS OF THE LIVER AND PANCREAS

LIVER FUNCTION TESTS

So-called liver function tests are not really function tests but a group of simultaneously performed laboratory tests designed to take a "biochemical snapshot" of the liver. Sometimes this group of tests is referred to as a liver profile. Similar profiles of tests are available for other organs such as the heart, lungs, and kidneys, and collectively these groups of tests are referred to as organ profiles.[1,2,IV]

1. In patients with clinical or laboratory findings of liver disease, request or review liver function tests.

In addition to clinical findings and abnormal blood tests, elevated urine bilirubin and urobilinogen may serve as clues to the presence of liver disease.[4] The composition of liver function tests may vary from one health care facility to another. An excellent combination of serum tests follows:

1. Aspartate aminotransferase (AST or SGOT)
2. Alanine aminotransferase (ALT or SGPT)
3. Alkaline phosphatase
4. Bilirubin, total and conjugated
5. Prothrombin time
6. Albumin and globulins by protein electrophoresis

Serum gamma-glutamyl transferase (GGT) and bile acids are two additional very sensitive tests for liver disease of any variety. The sensitivity of routine liver function tests for ruling out liver disease can be increased by measuring serum GGT and bile acids; however, these tests are not usually necessary.

Liver function tests are easier to understand and interpret if we view them according to the pathophysiologic derangements that cause the test results to become abnormal. Thus five pathophysiologic questions are useful to ask.[VI]

a. Is liver disease present or not? Measure all liver function tests.

Maximal sensitivity for detecting liver disease is achieved by performing all liver function tests at the same time. If all test results are normal, then it is unlikely that there is significant liver disease.

b. Is there liver cell injury and what is its severity? Measure serum transaminase levels: AST (SGOT) and ALT (SGPT).

Both AST (SGOT) and ALT (SGPT) are liver cell enzymes that are released into the blood following injury to the liver cell membranes, and significant elevations are characteristic of acute hepatitis. Elevation of serum transaminase levels correlates poorly with abnormal liver cell morphology by light microscopy. Remember that ALT (SGPT) tends to be higher than AST (SGOT) in viral hepatitis and that the reverse is true in alcoholic hepatitis. ALT (SGPT) has been used as a screening test for viral hepatitis.[3]

c. Is there cholestasis? Measure serum alkaline phosphatase and serum total and conjugated bilirubin.

Elevations of serum alkaline phosphatase and bilirubin are good tests for intrahepatic or extrahepatic obstruction, and serum alkaline phosphatase tends to be more sensitive than bilirubin. Elevation of serum GGT is another good test for cholestasis. GGT is a useful test to order when the patient has an elevated serum alkaline phosphatase and it is unclear whether the alkaline phosphatase is coming from liver or bone. GGT is high in liver disease but not in bone disease. Also, GGT can be useful in diagnosing liver disease in adolescence and pregnancy when the alkaline phosphatase cannot be used to assess the liver because it is high as a result of bone growth and the placenta, respectively. Serum bile acids are always elevated in cholestasis, but they are normal in the hereditary hyperbilirubinemias, such as Gilbert's disease. Cholesterol is also elevated in cholestasis. Cholestasis is characteristic of a metastatic infiltrate in the liver, as well as granulomatous infiltrates (tuberculosis, histoplasmosis, sarcoidosis) and hepatic abscesses.

In acute biliary obstruction of less than 24 hours' duration initial transaminase levels are frequently above 300 U/L. These values show a consistent dramatic reduction within the next 72 hours (mean AST [SGOT] fell from 339 to 97 U/L, and mean ALT [SGPT] fell from 527 to 221 U/L). Bilirubin levels fall less dramatically, and alkaline phosphatase levels are unpredictable. When these serial transaminase changes occur with absence of visualization of the biliary tract and bowel during cholescintigraphy, the diagnosis of acute biliary obstruction is almost certain.[5]

d. Are the metabolic functions of the liver compromised? Measure plasma prothrombin time and serum albumin (preferably by electrophoresis).

Depressed synthesis of proteins, especially serum albumin and the plasma coagulation factors, is a sensitive test for metabolic derangement of the liver. Measurement of serum albumin by protein electrophoresis is more accurate than dye-binding methods such as bromcresol green, and a plasma prothrombin time is a good way to assess plasma coagulation factors that are synthesized by the liver. In patients with hepatocellular damage, a low serum albumin suggests decreased protein synthesis and a significantly prolonged prothrombin time indicates a poor prognosis.

e. Is the disease process acute or chronic? Measure serum globulins (preferably by electrophoresis).

Most acute liver diseases do not cause significant elevations of serum globulins, but chronic liver diseases commonly show a polyclonal elevation of gamma globulins. Measurement of gamma globulins by protein electrophoresis is an excellent way to help in assessment of whether the liver disease is acute or chronic. For example, in chronic hepatitis and cirrhosis, one commonly sees a polyclonal gammopathy.

2.　If one or more test results are abnormal, then liver disease may be present. Analyze the pattern of abnormalities for clues concerning the type of liver disease and remember that false-positive test results may occur.

The best method for diagnosing liver disease is microscopic examination of a liver biopsy. Serum tests provide indirect information about hepatic pathophysiology. Significant elevations of serum transaminase (i.e., greater than 300 to 500 U/L) may indicate marked damage to liver cells and suggest acute hepatitis, although spikes of serum transaminase to high levels can also occur in chronic liver disease. Prominent elevations of alkaline phosphatase and bilirubin, especially conjugated bilirubin, suggest biliary obstruction. Significant depression of serum albumin and prolongation of plasma prothrombin time suggest serious metabolic derangement of the liver. Elevation of serum gamma globulins raises the possibility of chronic hepatitis or cirrhosis or both. Remember that there are tissue sources other than the liver for elevated serum transaminase and alkaline phosphatase levels. Transaminase elevations may originate in the heart, pancreas, and skeletal muscle, and alkaline phosphatase elevations may originate in the bone, intestines, and placenta.[1,2]

3.　If the liver function test results are all normal, then the liver is probably normal—the level of confidence is higher if serum GGT and bile acids are also normal.

Years ago, physicians used a normal bromsulphalein (BSP) excretion test to rule out liver disease, but this test has fallen into disuse because of anaphylactoid reactions and severe tissue irritation at sites of extravasation of the BSP. A safer excretion test using indocyanine green (ICG) is available but is little used. Moreover, normality of all routine liver function tests is pretty good evidence against liver disease, and if serum GGT and bile acids are also normal, the probability of liver disease is very low indeed, perhaps only about 1% to 2%. Still, a liver disorder can occasionally occur with normal liver function test results—a common example being fatty liver.

REFERENCES

1.　Chopra S, Griffin PH: Laboratory tests and diagnostic procedures in evaluation of liver disease. Am J Med 79:221, 1985.
2.　Helzberg JH, Spiro HM: "LFTs" test more than the liver. JAMA 256:3006, 1986.
3.　Jensen DM, Dickerson DD, Linderman MA, et al: Serum alanine aminotransferase levels and prevalence of hepatitis A, B, and delta in outpatients. Arch Intern Med 147:1734, 1987.
4.　Kupka T, Binder LS, Smith DA, et al: Accuracy of urine urobilinogen and bilirubin assays in predicting liver function abnormalities. Ann Emerg Med 16:1231, 1987.
5.　Patwardhan RV, Smith DJ, Farmelant MH: Serum transaminase levels and cholescintigraphic abnormalities in acute biliary obstruction. Arch Intern Med 147:1249, 1987.

ACUTE VIRAL HEPATITIS*

In the United States, about 60% of acute viral hepatitis is type B; about 20% is type A; and about 20% is type non-A, non-B. All these types of acute hepatitis may have a similar clinical picture. An important distinction is that hepatitis A does not cause chronic hepatitis, whereas hepatitis B and hepatitis non-A, non-B, do. Additional causes of acute viral hepatitis include Epstein-Barr virus, cytomegalovirus, and herpes virus. The diagnosis of acute viral hepatitis involves documentation of positive serologic tests for hepatitis A or hepatitis B in the context of the appropriate clinical and laboratory findings. Since there are no serologic tests for hepatitis non-A, non-B, the diagnosis rests on clinical findings and nonspecific laboratory test results. Hepatitis delta only occurs in patients who are already infected with hepatitis B. Clinical findings of acute hepatitis are typically constitutional and gastrointestinal.[2,3,6]

1. In patients with clinical findings and liver function test results of acute viral hepatitis, request serologic tests for hepatitis A and B, namely, anti-hepatitis A IgM antibody, hepatitis B surface antigen, and anti-hepatitis B core IgM antibody. Reserve hepatitis delta and hepatitis B e antigen testing for patients who are positive for hepatitis B.

There are no tests for hepatitis non-A, non-B, and testing for hepatitis delta should not be done unless the patient is determined to have hepatitis B and a deteriorating clinical condition caused by hepatitis. One other test for hepatitis A is anti-hepatitis A IgG antibody.[†] Its presence indicates a remote hepatitis A infection in the past. Several other tests for hepatitis B are available—anti-hepatitis B surface antibody, anti-hepatitis B core IgG antibody[†], hepatitis B e antigen, and anti-hepatitis B e antibody. These other tests for hepatitis B are only useful after it has been determined that a patient has hepatitis B, since they can help to answer three questions: (1) when has the infection resolved? (2) what is the risk that this patient may infect others? and (3) when has the infection become chronic?[6]

The serum AST (SGOT) and ALT (SGPT) are elevated from 500 to 5000 U/L or more, but levels less than 500 U/L may be seen in mild illness. Usually, the ALT (SGPT) exceeds the AST (SGOT). The magnitude of the transaminase elevation is not well correlated with the severity of liver damage. Serum bilirubin is commonly elevated from 5 to 20 mg/dl (85 to 342 μmol/L); levels above 30 mg/dl (513 μmol/L) suggest severe disease or hemolysis. Alkaline phosphatase is slightly elevated but may be markedly elevated in the presence of severe cholestasis. Serum gamma globulins may be slightly elevated: levels over 3.0 g/dl suggest chronic disease. Depression of serum albumin and a prolonged prothrombin time reflect impairment of liver protein synthesis and parallel the severity of the disease. Elevation of the prothrombin time beyond 20 seconds suggests the development of acute hepatic insufficiency.

The following clues concerning different varieties of viral hepatitis are helpful. Hepatitis A has fecal/oral transmission, a 20- to 37-day incubation

---

*Hepatitis A; hepatitis B; hepatitis non-A, non-B; hepatitis delta.

†Some laboratories may offer total anti-hepatitis A antibody and total anti-hepatitis B core antibody.

period, and up to a 45% prevalence in the U.S. population, whereas hepatitis B has percutaneous/venereal transmission, a 60- to 110-day incubation period, and up to a 5% to 15% prevalence in the U.S. population. Hepatitis non-A, non-B, has a percutaneous and probably a venereal mode of transmission and a 35- to 70-day incubation period. It accounts for 80% to 90% of posttransfusion hepatitis and 12% to 25% of sporadic hepatitis. Water-borne epidemics of hepatitis A and hepatitis non-A, non-B, have been reported, but not hepatitis B.[2]

2.   **Evaluate the serologic tests.**

VIRAL SEROLOGIC TESTS IN ACUTE HEPATITIS

TYPE OF HEPATITIS	DIAGNOSTIC SEROLOGIC TESTS RESULTS
Hepatitis A	Anti–hepatitis A IgM antibody *positive*
Hepatitis B	Hepatitis B surface antigen *positive* Anti–hepatitis B core IgM antibody *negative* *or* Hepatitis B surface antigen *positive* Anti–hepatitis B core IgM antibody *positive* *or* Hepatitis B surface antigen *negative* Anti–hepatitis B core IgM antibody *positive*
Hepatitis delta	Serologic tests for hepatitis B (as above) *positive* Anti–hepatitis delta antibody *positive*

In hepatitis A the initial antibody response is anti–hepatitis A IgM antibody, which appears at about 3½ weeks after exposure and falls off at about 12 weeks. Anti–hepatitis A IgG antibody appears at about 4 weeks and persists indefinitely, thus providing lifetime immunity. Therefore the presence of anti–hepatitis A IgM antibody indicates acute infection and the presence of anti–hepatitis A IgG antibody indicates remote infection in the past. There may be a period during a resolving infection when both of these antibodies are present simultaneously. Complications of hepatitis A are rare, and there is no evidence that infection with the hepatitis A virus results in a carrier state or chronic liver disease.[2]

In hepatitis B, hepatitis B surface antigen appears first at about 4 to 12 weeks after exposure, followed by anti–hepatitis B core IgM antibody a little later and anti–hepatitis B surface IgG antibody still later. There is a time period when hepatitis B surface antigen disappears and anti–hepatitis B surface IgG antibody has not yet appeared, when anti–hepatitis B core IgM antibody may be the only positive diagnostic test result. During the first 2 weeks of symptoms, hepatitis B surface antigen is more sensitive than the test for anti–hepatitis B core IgM antibody, but this is reversed 2 weeks after the onset of symptoms. The test for anti–hepatitis B core IgM antibody is better than the hepatitis B surface antigen test for detecting hepatitis B in the asymptomatic patient.[5] Of course, there may be times when hepatitis B surface antigen and anti–hepatitis B core

IgM antibody are present simultaneously or anti–hepatitis B core IgM antibody and anti–hepatitis B surface antibody IgG are present simultaneously. Almost all patients with acute hepatitis B have titers of anti–hepatitis B core IgM antibody at the time of initial examination, whereas chronic carriers of the virus have only low titers or no detectable anti–hepatitis B core IgM antibody at all.[4]

Hepatitis non-A, non-B, is a diagnosis of exclusion, since no tests for it are available. ALT (SGPT) is a good surrogate test.

Hepatitis delta is diagnosed by the presence of anti–hepatitis delta antibody. The usual clinical situation is that of a patient with chronic, asymptomatic, or acute hepatitis B who suddenly becomes markedly worse clinically. In some of these patients the level of hepatitis B antigenemia drops precipitously. However, even in these patients anti–hepatitis B core positivity remains. A characteristic biphasic aminotransferase elevation may result from the sequential infection of hepatitis B followed by hepatitis delta.[2,6]

3.   If hepatitis B surface antigen or anti-hepatitis B core IgM antibody or both are present, diagnose acute hepatitis B and request hepatitis B e antigen and anti-hepatitis B e antibody. If anti-hepatitis A IgM antibody is present, diagnose hepatitis A.

The presence of hepatitis B e antigen indicates patients who are very infectious, being much more likely to infect others than are patients who are simply hepatitis B surface antigen positive without e antigen. If anti–hepatitis B e antibody is present, it indicates that the hepatitis is beginning to resolve.[6]

4.   If diagnostic test results for hepatitis A, hepatitis B, and hepatitis delta are negative, consider other viruses that can cause hepatitis.

HEPATITIS NON-A, NON-B

Consider hepatitis non-A, non-B, in patients who have received transfusions of blood products. The disease may also occur sporadically. Since there are no specific serologic tests for hepatitis non-A, non-B, the diagnosis relies on clinical findings and surrogate tests, such as an elevated alanine aminotransferase (ALT or SGPT). Up to 40% of patients who develop hepatitis non-A, non-B, after transfusion develop chronic disease—many develop chronic active hepatitis and progress to cirrhosis.[2]

EPSTEIN-BARR HEPATITIS

Consider Epstein-Barr hepatitis (often part of the infectious mononucleosis syndrome) with these findings: nausea and vomiting, jaundice, and serum transaminase levels up to 500 U/L. The presence of heterophile antibodies or a rise in titer of specific antibodies to Epstein-Barr virus confirms the diagnosis.

CYTOMEGALOVIRUS HEPATITIS

Consider cytomegalovirus hepatitis (sometimes as part of an infectious mono-nucleosis syndrome without adenopathy or tonsillopharyngeal involvement) in patients with clinical and laboratory findings of mild acute hepatitis. Infection can be demonstrated by inoculation of appropriate tissue culture with urine or an increase in complement-fixation or indirect hemagglutination titers after an attack.

HERPES VIRUS HEPATITIS

Consider hepatitis caused by herpes simplex or varicella virus in patients with clinical and laboratory findings of acute hepatitis, often accompanied by typical skin lesions in immunocompromised patients. Presence of herpetic skin lesions demonstrable by a Tzanck test does not necessarily mean that the hepatitis is caused by herpes virus.

5.   After diagnosing acute viral hepatitis, begin therapy and monitor the patient's chemical and serologic (immunologic) test results.

For acute hepatitis A, there is no carrier state or possibility of chronic hepatitis , so serologic monitoring of these patients is not necessary.

For acute hepatitis B, serologic monitoring is mandatory. Anti-hepatitis B core IgG antibody appears before hepatitis B surface IgG antibody and persists throughout life. It is the best single marker of exposure to hepatitis B virus. For determining when the infection has resolved, test for hepatitis B surface IgG antibody monthly. If by 6 months after the acute episode the patient is no longer hepatitis B surface antigen positive and is anti-hepatitis B surface IgG antibody positive, then the patient has eliminated the virus and a full and complete recovery has occurred. Such a patient will have no chronic sequelae and can no longer infect others. After 1 to 23 months anti-hepatitis B surface antibody may be lost, but anti-hepatitis B core antibody always persists.[7] For patients who are hepatitis B e antigen positive, test for anti-hepatitis B e antibody monthly, since *the appearance of anti-hepatitis B e antibody will indicate when the patient is less infectious to others.* In patients who do not develop anti-hepatitis B surface IgG antibody, the finding of two positive hepatitis B surface antigen results 6 months or more apart indicates chronic hepatitis (about 10% of acute hepatitis B patients develop chronic hepatitis). If there is no clinical and laboratory evidence of hepatitis, the patient is termed a "chronic carrier" (more often in men than women). If laboratory or biopsy evidence of hepatitis is present, the diagnosis is termed "chronic persistent hepatitis" or "chronic active hepatitis," depending on the histologic findings.[6]

The ALT (SGPT) is a good test to follow the course of acute viral hepatitis, because it is often the last test to return to normal.

6.   In patients with acute viral hepatitis, in addition to abnormal liver function tests, the following abnormal laboratory test results may occur:

HEMATOLOGY

- Mild transient anemia; rarely aplastic anemia
- Mild transient leukopenia with a relative lymphocytosis and atypical lymphocytes; a leukocytosis can occur in fulminant hepatitis
- Thrombocytopenia in fulminant disease

CHEMISTRY

- Hypoglycemia, often mild and insignificant, but profound hypoglycemia can occur in fulminant hepatitis
- Hyperuricemia related to hepatocellular damage
- Hyperamylasemia with concurrent pancreatitis
- Elevated lactate dehydrogenase (LD) from hepatocellular damage
- Hypocholesterolemia from depressed liver synthesis; degree of depression parallels severity of hepatitis

REFERENCES

1. Cutler P: Jaundice and pain (acute hepatitis). In Cutler P: Problem Solving in Clinical Medicine: From Data to Diagnosis, 2nd ed. Baltimore, Williams & Wilkins, 1985, p 397.
2. Gastroenterology Subspecialty Committee: Medical Knowledge Self-Assessment Program VIII. Gastroenterology. Philadelphia, American College of Physicians, 1988, p 428.
3. Holt JT, Arvan DA: Acute viral hepatitis. In Griner PF, Panzer RJ, Greenland P: Clinical Diagnosis and the Laboratory: Logical Strategies for Common Medical Problems. Chicago, Year Book Medical Publishers, Inc, 1986, p 270.
4. Lemon SM: What is the role of testing for IgM antibody to core antigen of hepatitis B virus? Mayo Clin Proc 63:201, 1988.
5. Lindsay KL, Nizze JA, Koretz R, et al: Diagnostic usefulness of testing for anti-HBc IgM in acute hepatitis B. Hepatology 6:1325, 1986.
6. Neff JC: Immunological (serological) diagnosis of viral hepatitis. University Reference Laboratories Inc, Laboratory Update, January-February, 1987.
7. Zito DR, Gurdak RG, Tucker FL, et al: Hepatitis B virus serology: Loss of antibody to surface antigen. Am J Clin Pathol 88:229, 1987.

FATTY LIVER AND ALCOHOLIC HEPATITIS

In the United States, about 10 million people are problem drinkers, and, of these, 6 million are alcoholics. Liver disease is a common manifestation of this disorder. The strategy for the diagnosis and management of alcoholic liver disease involves a combination of clinical findings, liver function tests, and other procedures. Histologic findings on liver biopsy vary from fatty liver to alcoholic hepatitis and cirrhosis. In developed countries alcohol-related liver disease is the most common cause for cirrhosis, and, even when consumption is corrected for body weight, women are more susceptible than men. Clinical findings of fatty liver and alcoholic hepatitis vary from none to those of acute hepatic failure.[1-5]

1. In patients with clinical findings and liver function test results of fatty liver or alcoholic hepatitis, to accurately diagnose the lesion, consider obtaining a needle biopsy of the liver.

Alcohol abuse causes three main pathologic lesions: fatty liver, alcoholic hepatitis, and cirrhosis. Patients may have clinical features particular to each of these lesions or mixed clinical findings caused by combinations of these pathologic lesions. Often, the patient can be treated without a liver biopsy;

however, if the clinical findings are severe enough to require an accurate diagnosis, a biopsy is appropriate.

In fatty liver, the asparate aminotransferase (AST or SGOT) may be normal to modestly elevated, up to 400 U/L (ratio of AST to ALT is often $\geq 2{:}1$). Serum bilirubin elevation to 5 mg/dl (85 μmol/L) may occur with mild elevation of alkaline phosphatase, although occasionally intense cholestasis develops. Serum albumin and globulins are abnormal in about 25% of patients, and serum gamma-glutamyl transferase (GGT) is usually elevated.

In alcoholic hepatitis, the leukocyte count is elevated and may exceed 30,000 to 40,000/mm³. Regarding the liver, the AST (SGOT) may be elevated to 600 U/L, and AST (SGOT) is higher than ALT (SGPT). Frequently, the AST (SGOT) is more than twice as high as ALT (SGPT). Serum bilirubin and alkaline phosphatase may be moderately elevated, and a small percentage of patients develops a cholestatic picture with high bilirubin (up to 30 mg/dl [513 μmol/L]) and high alkaline phosphatase as the predominant abnormalities. Prolongation of the prothrombin time, hypoalbuminemia, and hyperglobulinemia may be present.

2. Evaluate the tests.

The best method for the diagnosis of fatty liver and alcoholic hepatitis is microscopic examination of a liver biopsy.

3. If a liver biopsy shows fatty change of the large droplet variety, it is consistent with the fatty liver of alcohol abuse.

Large droplet fatty change is not specific for alcohol abuse but may be seen in other conditions, such as jejunoileal bypass for obesity or diabetes mellitus. The lesion may also be caused by corticosteroids and antimetabolites (methotrexate). Alcoholic fatty liver is reversible if the patient stops drinking.

4. If a liver biopsy shows hepatocellular necrosis with infiltration by polymorphonuclear leukocytes, it is consistent with alcoholic hepatitis.

The essential feature of alcoholic hepatitis is hepatocellular necrosis and infiltration by polymorphonuclear leukocytes. Alcoholic hyaline may be present or absent. Fibrosis may be present within the lobule and around the central vein where it can cause obstruction of blood flow and portal hypertension. Patients with alcoholic hepatitis may develop the hepatorenal syndrome—rising serum urea nitrogen and creatinine indicate a poor prognosis, and these patients may develop cirrhosis. Amiodarone toxicity can simulate alcoholic hepatitis.[5]

REFERENCES

1. Cutler P: Jaundice and pain (acute hepatitis). In Cutler P: Problem Solving in Clinical Medicine: From Data to Diagnosis, 2nd ed. Baltimore, Williams & Wilkins, 1985, p 397.
2. Gastroenterology Subspecialty Committee: Medical Knowledge Self-Assessment Program VIII. Gastroenterology. Philadelphia, American College of Physicians, 1988, p 428.
3. Lieber CS: Alcohol and the liver: 1984 update. Hepatology 4:1243, 1984.

4. Lieber CS: Biochemical and molecular basis of alcohol-induced injury to liver and other tissues. N Engl J Med 319:1639, 1988.
5. Sherlock S: Disease of the Liver and Biliary System, 7th ed. Oxford, England, Blackwell Scientific Publications, 1985.

ACUTE NONVIRAL, NONALCOHOLIC HEPATITIS*

Acute nonviral, nonalcoholic hepatitis includes a number of disorders that may be confused with acute viral hepatitis. Some of these are common, such as drug-related hepatitis and heart-failure hepatitis, whereas others are more unusual, such as hepatic vein–occlusion hepatitis. They are all important. The strategy for diagnosing these other acute hepatitides is to rule out the acute viral and alcoholic hepatitides and then to recognize the clinical findings, laboratory test results, and results of other studies that typically occur in each of the nonviral, nonalcoholic acute hepatitides. The clinical findings may resemble those of acute viral hepatitis.[1,3,5]

In patients with clinical findings and liver function test results of acute hepatitis, in whom acute viral hepatitis and alcoholic hepatitis have been excluded, consider hepatitis caused by drugs, toxins, heart failure, hepatic vein occlusion, and Reye's syndrome.

All of these kinds of hepatitis may be confused with acute viral hepatitis because of similar clinical and laboratory findings, such as an elevated serum transaminase. Since there are few specific diagnostic tests, diagnosis often depends on a careful analysis of the history, physical examination, laboratory findings, and results of other studies.

DRUG-INDUCED HEPATITIS

Consider drug-induced hepatitis in patients with these findings: clinical and chemical evidence of acute hepatitis, onset of hepatitis 2 to 6 weeks after starting drug therapy (but may occur as early as the first day or not until 6 months later). The hepatitis may progress even after drug withdrawal, and failure to withdraw the offending drug can cause death. Almost any drug may rarely cause hepatitis. Older patients and women appear more susceptible. Idiosyncratic or unpredictable causes of drug hepatitis include anesthetics (halothane, chloroform); tranquilizers (phenothiazines, haloperidol, diazepam, chlordiazepoxide); antidepressants (iproniazid, tricyclics); anticonvulsants (phenytoin, carbamazepine); antiarthritics (gold, allopurinol, probenecid, non-steroidal antiinflammatory drugs); all the hypoglycemics; antithyroidal drugs; some antimicrobials (clindamycin, isoniazid, rifampin, sulfonamides); cardiac drugs (methyldopa, quinidine, procainamide); and most cancer chemotherapeutic agents. Halothane hepatitis is more common in overweight women with repeated

---

*Includes discussion of drug-induced hepatitis, toxic hepatitis, heart-failure hepatitis, hepatic vein–occlusion hepatitis, and Reye's syndrome.

exposures. Patients may have fever, malaise, eosinophilia, elevated serum transaminase and bilirubin, depressed albumin, and prolonged prothrombin time. The histologic findings may resemble viral hepatitis, and granulomata are frequently seen. Predictable causes of drug hepatitis include acetaminophen; more than 25 g orally will cause profound acute hepatitis with hepatocellular necrosis in most persons. N-acetylcysteine can reverse the process if given within 8 hours of an acetaminophen overdose, and treatment is still indicated as late as 24 hours after ingestion.[3,5,6]

TOXIC HEPATITIS

Consider toxic hepatitis in patients with severe acute hepatitis exposed to poisoning, such as carbon tetrachloride or the wild mushroom *Amanita phalloides*. The mortality is high.[5]

HEART-FAILURE HEPATITIS

Consider heart-failure hepatitis in patients with elevated serum transaminase levels up to thousands of units per liter and sometimes jaundice. These patients may have marked hypotension, shock, or severe acute congestive heart failure.[1,4]

HEPATIC VEIN-OCCLUSION HEPATITIS

Consider hepatic vein–occlusion hepatitis (Budd-Chiari syndrome) in patients with these findings: acute abdominal pain, tender hepatomegaly, ascites, and liver function tests consistent with acute hepatitis. Causes include myeloproliferative disorders, bone marrow transplants, birth control pills, food contaminated with pyrrolizidine alkaloids. Most cases progress to death from hepatic failure and variceal bleeding.[5]

REYE'S SYNDROME

Consider Reye's syndrome in children with these findings: sudden onset of intractable vomiting a few days after a viral illness, history of aspirin ingestion, cloudy sensorium, seizures, coma, enlarged liver, hypoglycemia, and abnormal liver function tests. Liver biopsy reveals fatty change of the microvesicular variety with little or no inflammation.[2]

REFERENCES

1. Cohen JA, Kaplan MM: Left-sided heart failure presenting as hepatitis. Gastroenterology 74:583, 1978.
2. DeVivo DC: Reye syndrome. Neurol Clin 3:95, 1985.
3. Gastroenterology Subspecialty Committee: Medical Knowledge Self-Assessment Program VIII. Gastroenterology. Philadelphia, American College of Physicians, 1988, p 430.
4. Kubo SH, Walter BA, John DHA et al: Liver function abnormalities in chronic heart failure. Influence of systemic hemodynamics. Arch Intern Med 147:1227, 1987.
5. Sherlock DS: Diseases of the Liver and Biliary System, 7th ed. Oxford, England, Blackwell Scientific Publications, 1985.

6. Smilkstein MJ, Knapp GL, Kulig KW, et al: Efficacy of oral *N*-acetylcysteine in the treatment of acetaminophen overdose. N Engl J Med 319:1557, 1988.

CHRONIC PERSISTENT AND CHRONIC ACTIVE HEPATITIS

Chronic persistent hepatitis and chronic active hepatitis are varieties of chronic inflammation of the liver characterized by chronic inflammation of the portal triads. Whereas chronic persistent hepatitis is usually benign, chronic active hepatitis can progress to macronodular cirrhosis and liver failure. The diagnostic strategy involves determining whether chronic hepatitis exists, and if it does, whether it is chronic persistent or chronic active hepatitis. An etiology must be sought, so that proper therapy can be initiated, especially if the diagnosis is chronic active hepatitis.[1-3,6]

1.   In patients with clinical findings and liver function test results of chronic hepatitis, request serologic tests for hepatitis B (i.e., hepatitis B surface antigen and anti-hepatitis B core IgG antibody*), and, to accurately diagnose the lesion, consider obtaining a needle biopsy of the liver.

Chronic hepatitis may be caused by viruses, drugs, unknown factors, and unusual metabolic diseases such as alpha₁-antitrypsin deficiency and Wilson's disease.

When chronic hepatitis follows acute hepatitis, persistence longer than 6 months can be used to make the diagnosis. Sometimes, however, the disease begins insidiously, or the problem may surface when an apparently healthy person is found to have an elevated serum transaminase level by laboratory screening or a positive test for hepatitis B is discovered when the person attempts to donate blood. In these latter instances, a polyclonal gammopathy on serum protein electrophoresis may be a clue that you are dealing with a chronic hepatitis.

In chronic persistent hepatitis, serum transaminase levels may vary from normal to moderately elevated (40 to 200 U/L) and the values may fluctuate. Serum alkaline phosphatase and bilirubin may be normal to slightly elevated, and serum albumin and the plasma prothrombin time are usually normal. Moderate elevations of gamma globulins up to about 2.0 g/dl may be seen. Antinuclear antibodies (ANAs) are usually absent, and the lupus erythematosus (LE) cell preparation is negative.

In chronic active hepatitis, serum transaminase elevations greater than 400 U/L are common with possible elevations to much higher levels, usually occurring during exacerbations of the disease. Serum alkaline phosphatase may be elevated, and bilirubin levels of 3 to 10 mg/dl (51 to 171 μmol/L) or more commonly occur. Depressed serum albumin and a prolonged prothrombin time may occur, and the degree of abnormality parallels the severity of the disease process. Serum globulins are commonly elevated and may reach the 3 to

---

*Some laboratories may offer total anti-hepatitis B core antibody.

7 g/dl range. ANAs are frequently found, and the LE cell preparation is positive in 10% to 20% of patients.

2. Evaluate the tests.

The best method for the diagnosis of chronic hepatitis and the differentiation of chronic persistent hepatitis and chronic active hepatitis is microscopic examination of a liver biopsy.

With the exception of alpha$_1$-antitrypsin deficiency, the cause of chronic active hepatitis cannot be determined from the histology. PAS-positive material in hepatocytes after diastase treatment is characteristic of alpha$_1$-antitrypsin deficiency. Copper stains for Wilson's disease are often unreliable.

VIRAL SEROLOGIC TESTS IN CHRONIC HEPATITIS

TYPE OF HEPATITIS	DIAGNOSTIC SEROLOGIC TEST RESULTS
Hepatitis B	Hepatitis B surface antigen *positive* Anti–hepatitis B core IgG antibody *positive*

3. If the liver biopsy shows chronic active hepatitis, determine its etiology so that appropriate therapy may be chosen. If serologic test results are positive for hepatitis B, request tests for anti–hepatitis B core IgM antibody, hepatitis B e antigen, and hepatitis delta, if appropriate.

About 20% of cases of chronic active hepatitis are associated with and probably caused by hepatitis B with or without superimposed hepatitis delta infection. In contrast to patients with acute hepatitis B who have high titers of anti–hepatitis B core IgM antibody at the time of initial examination, chronic carriers of the virus have low titers or no detectable anti–hepatitis B core IgM antibody at all. However, chronic carriers with the antibody are more likely to have active liver disease, hepatitis B e antigen positivity, and detectable viremia (hepatitis B virus DNA positive by DNA-DNA hybridization).[1,5] Chronic active hepatitis, which has no serologic markers, may also follow hepatitis non-A, non-B, so a history of transfusion is important. Hepatitis A does not cause chronic active hepatitis.

Drugs that can cause chronic active hepatitis include amiodarone, dantrolene, isoniazid, methyldopa, nitrofurantoin, oxyphenisatin, perhexilene maleate, phenytoin, propylthiouracil, and sulfonamides. Long-term use of acetaminophen, aspirin, and ethanol may occasionally cause the syndrome.[x]

Wilson's disease and alpha$_1$-antitrypsin deficiency may be seen as chronic active hepatitis. In many patients the etiology is unknown. A number of these patients (usually young women) will exhibit clinical features and serologic findings of autoimmune chronic active hepatitis (formerly lupoid hepatitis), such as positive antinuclear antibodies (ANAs), a positive lupus erythematosus (LE) cell preparation, double-stranded DNA antibody, smooth muscle antibody, and a polyclonal hypergammaglobulinemia with the IgG fraction predominating. A history of transfusion is important, since hepatitis non-A, non-B, which accounts for 80% to 90% of posttransfusion hepatitis, has a high tendency to become chronic.

Patients with chronic active hepatitis may develop cirrhosis. Hepatocellular carcinoma is an additional complication that can develop in patients with chronic hepatitis B.[4]

4. If the liver biopsy shows chronic persistent hepatitis, reassure the patient and continue observation.

For chronic persistent hepatitis related to hepatitis B, regular monitoring (about every 6 months) is mandatory to determine whether hepatitis B and e antigens persist or whether these antigens are replaced by anti–hepatitis B and e antibodies, in which case the patient is cured. About 15% of patients with chronic hepatitis B develop antibodies and are cured each year.

5. In patients with chronic active hepatitis, in addition to abnormal liver function tests, the following additional abnormal laboratory test results may occur:

HEMATOLOGY

- Anemia
- Leukopenia
- Thrombocytopenia
- Hypoglycemia related to destruction of hepatic tissue

REFERENCES

1. Alter HJ (ed): Hepatitis. Semin Liv Dis 6:1, 1986.
2. Bentch HL: Swelling of the abdomen (chronic hepatitis). In Cutler P: Problem Solving in Clinical Medicine: From Data to Diagnosis, 2nd ed. Baltimore, Williams & Wilkins, 1985, p 527.
3. Czaja AJ: Current problems in the diagnosis and management of chronic active hepatitis. Mayo Clin Proc 56:311, 1981.
4. Gastroenterology Subspecialty Committee: Medical Knowledge Self-Assessment Program VIII. Gastroenterology. Philadelphia, American College of Physicians, 1988, p 430.
5. Lemon SM: What is the role of testing for IgM antibody to core antigen of hepatitis B virus? Mayo Clin Proc 63:201, 1988.
6. Vyas GN, Deinstag JL, Hoofnagle JH (eds): Viral Hepatitis and Liver Disease. Orlando, Grune & Stratton, 1984.

ACUTE PANCREATITIS

More than 90% of patients with acute pancreatitis have alcohol abuse or cholelithiasis as an underlying cause. Additional conditions that predispose to acute pancreatitis include hypercalcemia, hypertriglyceridemia, liver trauma, penetrating peptic ulcer, abdominal surgery, endoscopic retrograde pancreatography, drugs (thiazide and related diuretics, furosemide, estrogens, oral contraceptives, corticosteroids, azathioprine, sulfonamides, tetracycline, L-asparaginase, 6-mercaptopurine, methyldopa, procainamide), pregnancy, infections (mumps, hepatitis, other viruses, ascaris, mycoplasma), vasculitis, obstruction of the ampulla of Vater, renal failure and postrenal transplantation, and as an inherited autosomal dominant trait. Many patients develop elevated serum amylase levels after endoscopic retrograde cholangiopancreatography, but clinical pancreatitis occurs in less than 1% of patients after this procedure. The diagnosis depends on a gestalt of clinical, radiographic, and laboratory features, and for most cases, the best method for diagnosis (histologic demonstration of pancreatic inflammation) is not available. At least 95% of patients experience excruciating midepigastric pain, which typically radiates directly through to the back. Mortality in patients with acute pancreatitis is about 10%.[1,2,5-8]

1. In patients with clinical findings of acute pancreatitis, request a complete blood count (CBC); serum creatinine, amylase, lipase, and calcium; urinary creatinine and amylase; liver function tests; and triglycerides. If there is a pleural effusion, consider needle aspiration and measurement of pleural fluid amylase.

A CBC will detect the leukocytosis of pancreatitis, and serum amylase and serum lipase will detect the characteristic elevations of these enzymes in the blood. Serum creatinine, urinary creatinine, and urinary amylase enable one to detect renal failure as well as calculate the ratio of amylase clearance to creatinine clearance. Liver function tests are useful to detect associated biliary obstruction or hepatitis or both, and serum calcium and triglycerides can detect underlying causal factors.

2. If the clinical, radiographic, and laboratory findings are consistent with acute pancreatitis, the diagnosis is supported with a level of confidence that depends on the appropriateness of all the data.

The leukocyte count is frequently elevated in the range of 10,000 to 30,000 cells/mm^3, and the sedimentation rate will often be elevated to 30 mm/hr or more. Acute-phase reactants will be increased.

Serum and urine amylase levels tend to become elevated during the first 2 to 3 hours after the onset of pancreatitis, and, in mild to moderately severe attacks, they return to normal after 2 to 10 days. Amylase levels more than three times the upper limit of normal are almost always caused by pancreatitis.[1] The urine amylase level may be the last to return to normal. More prolonged elevation is encountered with more severe pancreatitis or when there has been recrudescence of the acute process during recovery. Elevations beyond 3 or 4 weeks are not uncommonly caused by pancreatic pseudocyst or pancreatic cancer.

The specificity of serum amylase as a test for acute pancreatitis is rather low, especially with values that are slightly elevated. A number of other conditions can be associated with elevations of serum amylase to these levels, such as renal failure, diabetic ketoacidosis, common bile duct obstruction, peptic ulcer, postgastric resection, intestinal obstruction, mesenteric thrombosis, peritonitis, salivary gland disease, chronic alcoholism, burns, malignant tumors, gynecologic disorders, and opiate administration. Serum amylase levels that are very elevated usually mean acute pancreatitis, and there is often an associated biliary tract disorder. The triad of elevated serum amylase, serum glucose, and blood leukocytes adds greater credence to the diagnosis of acute pancreatitis than elevation of serum amylase alone. Hyperamylasemia up to 1000 U/L or greater can occur in anorexia nervosa and bulimia: the cause is elevated salivary-type isoamylase and not pancreatitis. In patients with anorexia nervosa and bulimia, if serum lipase and pancreatic isoamylase levels are normal, pancreatitis is ruled out.[3]

The elevation of serum lipase is less sensitive but more specific as a test for acute pancreatitis than elevated serum amylase. Approximately 75% of patients with acute pancreatitis will have an elevated serum amylase, 65% an elevated lipase, and 85% an elevation of either one. Absence of elevation of either enzyme permits us to exclude acute pancreatitis with greater confidence because the combined sensitivity is greater than that for serum amylase alone. Usually, serum amylase increases before lipase, but occasionally the reverse occurs.[VI]

The specificity of serum lipase as a test for acute pancreatitis can be useful in distinguishing whether an elevated serum amylase is caused by acute inflammation of the parotid glands or acute pancreatitis. Serum amylase can be elevated in both of these disorders, whereas serum lipase is not elevated in inflammation of the parotid glands.

An elevated amylase/creatinine clearance ratio (reference interval: 1% to 4%) as a result of defective proximal tubular reabsorption of amylase occurs in many patients with clear-cut acute pancreatitis; however, about one third of patients with proven acute pancreatitis have amylase/creatinine clearance ratios that are not increased during the acute course of illness. Also, an increased amylase/creatinine clearance ratio is not specific for acute pancreatitis and can occur in patients with burns, diabetic ketoacidosis, acute defective tubular function, severe renal insufficiency, duodenal perforation, and pancreatic cancer. Therefore the amylase/creatinine clearance ratio is not a good test to diagnose acute pancreatitis.[VI]

An elevated serum amylase level in the presence of a urine amylase that is not elevated suggests macroamylasemia (polymerization of amylase or amylase bound to immunoglobin). Persons with macroamylasemia are usually well and do not have acute pancreatitis. The diagnosis may be confirmed by a low amylase/creatinine clearance ratio (below lower reference limit: <1.0%) despite normal renal function.[4]

Liver function test results can detect biliary obstruction as well as hepatitis of either viral or alcoholic etiology, and serum calcium and triglycerides can detect hypercalcemia or hypertriglyceridemia as associated causal factors. The presence on admission of a serum bilirubin above 2.3 mg/dl (40 μmol/L), a gamma-glutamyl transferase (GGT) above 250 U/L, an alkaline phosphatase (AP) above 225 U/L, and an age of 70 years or greater is highly predictive of common bile duct stones.[5] Hypertriglyceridemia (often above 1000 mg/dl [11.3 mmol/L]) may be seen in acute pancreatitis, and a history of drug ingestion is very important (e.g., women taking oral contraceptives). If hyperlipidemia is accompanied by acute hemolysis, jaundice, and alcoholic fatty change of the liver, the combination is called Zieve's syndrome.

Although a high pleural fluid amylase may occur in effusions in various diseases, absence of amylase in such an effusion is evidence against a diagnosis of acute pancreatitis.

3. If the serum amylase and lipase are normal, acute pancreatitis is possible but not probable.

Elevated levels of serum amylase and lipase are not perfectly sensitive for acute pancreatitis, and it is unfortunate but true that fatal acute pancreatitis can occur even when serum amylase values are not elevated. Reported sensitivities of serum amylase as a test for acute pancreatitis vary from 45% to 95%. Cases of acute pancreatitis related to excessive alcohol intake may have serum amylase values about two to four times normal. At this time, there are no definitive laboratory tests that can diagnose acute pancreatitis in the presence of normal serum amylase and lipase.

4. In patients with acute pancreatitis, the following additional abnormal laboratory test results may occur:

HEMATOLOGY

- Elevated hemoglobin and hematocrit caused by hemoconcentration but sometimes a decreased hemoglobin and hematocrit; possible hemolytic anemia
- Depressed platelet count with disseminated intravascular coagulation
- Moderately decreased PO_2 and moderately decreased O_2 saturation

CHEMISTRY

- Hyperglycemia
- Hyperuricemia, possibly from necrotic pancreatic tissue
- Mild hypokalemia
- Hypocalcemia related to decreased parathyroid hormone, increased thyrocalcitonin, decreased albumin; and calcium combining with free fatty acids
- Hypoalbuminemia
- Elevated creatine kinase and lactate dehydrogenase, possibly from necrotic pancreatic tissue
- Elevated transaminase (AST or SGOT) and other liver function tests caused by associated alcoholic liver disease; AST (SGOT) may also be released from necrotic pancreatic tissue

REFERENCES

1. Gastroenterology Subspecialty Committee: Medical Knowledge Self-Assessment Program VIII. Gastroenterology. Philadelphia, American College of Physicians, 1988, p 425.
2. Grendell JH, Egan J: Acute pancreatitis (Medical Staff Conference). West J Med 146:598, 1987.
3. Humpries LL, Adams LJ, Eckfeldt JH, et al: Hyperamylasemia in patients with eating disorders. Ann Intern Med 106:50, 1987.
4. Kleinman DS, O'Brien JF: Macroamylase. Mayo Clin Proc 61:669, 1986.
5. Neoptolemos JP, London N, Bailey I, et al: The role of clinical and biochemical criteria and endoscopic retrograde cholangiopancreatography in the urgent diagnosis of common bile duct stones in acute pancreatitis. Surgery 100:732, 1986.
6. Pestana C: Sudden upper abdominal pain (acute pancreatitis). In Cutler P: Problem Solving in Clinical Medicine: From Data to Diagnosis. Baltimore, Williams & Wilkins, 1985, p 377.
7. Spechler SJ: How much can we know about acute pancreatitis? Ann Intern Med 102:704, 1985.
8. Stoler MA, Arvan DA: Acute pancreatitis. In Griner PF, Panzer RJ, Greenland P: Clinical Diagnosis and the Laboratory: Logical Strategies for Common Medical Problems. Chicago, Year Book Medical Publishers, Inc, 1986, p 297.

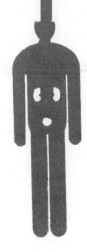

CHAPTER 7

98

URINARY TRACT DISORDERS

THE URINALYSIS

From the earliest times, the urinalysis has been regarded as an important indicator of an individual's state of health. This probably relates to the ease with which urine may be obtained and the patient's willingness to provide a urine specimen. A 1981 survey of medical practice by internists in the United States revealed that a urinalysis was performed in approximately 32% of patient encounters. It is perhaps the most frequently performed screening test. Traditionally, the urinalysis has been divided into macroscopic and microscopic examinations. Newer developments in dipstick technology and automation may make the microscopic examination unnecessary in some testing situations.[3,5]

The traditional macroscopic examination consists of a description of the urine, including its color and specific gravity. The usual dipstick provides a semiquantitative estimation of pH, glucose, protein, hemoglobin, ketones, bilirubin, and urobilinogen. Recently, two new dipstick tests have been added, the nitrite test and the leukocyte esterase test. Both of these new tests are designed to detect the presence of urinary tract infections. Gram-negative urinary bacteria reduce nitrates to nitrites, and urine polymorphonuclear leukocytes release leukocyte esterase.[5]

The microscopic examination is done by centrifuging 10 ml of urine at 2000 rpm for 5 minutes at about $450 \times g$ and resuspending the sediment in 1 ml. Under high power, erythrocytes, leukocytes, and renal epithelial cells are counted in 10 representative fields. Bacteria and yeasts are noted. Crystals are reported if their number is unusually large or they are abnormal. If casts are present, they are identified, and the number of casts per low-power field in 10 fields is reported. With the introduction of the nitrite and leukocyte esterase tests to detect bacteria and leukocytes in the urine, there have been a number of studies to determine whether it is necessary to perform a labor-intensive microscopic examination of the urinary sediment if all dipstick tests are completely negative.[IV]

1. In screening, request a urinalysis* using a dipstick (including the nitrite test and leukocyte esterase test). If all dipstick tests are negative, omit microscopic examination of the sediment.

---

*In the routine health-care setting, the urinalysis may be compromised by a poorly collected specimen, delays in testing, lack of standardization of procedures, and lack of proficiency by the examiner. Microscopic examination of the sediment is particularly vulnerable to these poor practices. If medically reliable information is to be obtained, emphasis must be placed on proper collection of a fresh specimen, which is quickly tested by a competent examiner using standardized and controlled techniques.

99

In patients with clinical findings of urinary tract disease, obtain a complete urinalysis—dipstick and microscopic examination of the sediment—regardless of the dipstick results.

In patients admitted to a general medicine ward, a urinalysis revealed abnormalities in 57%. In the general population it is much lower: 2.5% of men undergoing routine health screening were found to have hematuria; approximately 5% of women of childbearing age were found to have significant bacteriuria; and proteinuria is present in 0.6% to 5.8% of adults and diabetes in about 1.3%. Overall, in a survey of patients in general practice, 11% of males and 18% of females had urinary abnormalities, most of which were detected by dipstick testing rather than by microscopy.[4] In routine dipstick analysis of 21,000 presumably healthy, employed adults, 10% of subjects had at least one abnormality (12% of women and 8% of men), with increasing prevalence with age. The most common abnormality in women was hematuria (8.1%) and in men proteinuria (4.9%), but the rates for glucosuria (0.6%) and ketone bodies (0.4% to 0.5%) were about the same for both sexes.[2] Another study suggests that in spite of the high prevalence (34%) of abnormalities on routine hospital admission urinalysis, the impact on patient care is small and there is little justification for ordering the test for all patients admitted to the hospital.[1] A practical approach appears advisable—wide application of urine dipstick technology is an effective test to detect covert pyuria, hematuria, and proteinuria as a part of a routine physical examination. The test is inexpensive and can detect diseases that cause serious morbidity. A negative result is also useful as baseline information.[8] A urine dipstick test may even be useful to detect sexually transmitted disease in the male.[7] Pregnant women should have regular urinalyses with urine cultures if pyuria is noted.[6] Compared with 5 leukocytes per high power (HPF), the leukocyte esterase test has a sensitivity of 78% to 99% and a specificity of 69% to 99%. If read at 5 minutes, not 1 to 2 minutes, the sensitivity for more than 3 leukocytes per HPF is 100%.[5]

Recently, it has been shown that if the extended dipstick tests (including nitrite and leukocyte esterase) are negative, the false-negative results by microscopic examination are only about 1% to 2.9%. Clearly, the microscopic examination is the most time-consuming and costly part of the urinalysis, and it can be omitted in the context of screening for urinary tract disorders, if all the dipstick test results are negative. However, when there are clinical findings, the microscopic examination should be performed regardless of the dipstick results.[5]

2. Interpret urinalysis test results in the context of clinical findings.

Positive test results, either macroscopic or microscopic, should always be explored further. The presence of glucose, protein, or hemoglobin may be a clue to serious disease or may represent a benign finding that, once explained, can be disregarded. Erythrocytes, leukocytes, epithelial cells, bacteria, casts, and other findings in the urinary sediment may constitute key information in diagnosing a urinary tract disorder. The problems that follow discuss the workup of glucosuria, proteinuria, and hemoglobinuria, as well as the use of urinalysis in the diagnosis of urinary tract infection in women.

REFERENCES

1. Akin BV, Hubbell FA, Frye EB, et al: Efficacy of routine admission urinalysis. Am J Med 82:719, 1987.
2. Carel RS, Silverberg DS, Kaminsky R, et al: Routine urinalysis (dipstick) findings in mass screening of healthy adults. Clin Chem 33:2106, 1987.
3. Carlson DA, Statland BE: Automated urinalysis. Clin Lab Med 8:449, 1988.
4. Is routine urinalysis worthwhile? Lancet 1:747, 1988.
5. Kiel DP, Moskowitz MA: The urinalysis: A critical appraisal. Med Clin North Am 71:607, 1987.
6. Komaroff AL: Urinalysis and urine culture in women with dysuria. In Sox HC (ed): Common Diagnostic Tests. Use and Interpretation. Philadelphia, American College of Physicians, 1987, p 238.
7. Sadof MD, Woods ER, Emans SJ: Dipstick leukocyte esterase activity in first-catch urine specimens. A useful screening test for detecting sexually transmitted disease in the adolescent male. JAMA 258:1932, 1987.
8. Sodeman TM: Urinalysis and urine culture in women with dysuria. In Glenn GC (ed): Blue Cross/Blue Shield Association Guidelines Based on Common Diagnostic Tests. Use and Interpretation. Skokie, IL, College of American Pathologists, 1988, p 15.

GLUCOSURIA

Glucosuria usually occurs when the serum level is more than 180 to 200 mg/dl (9.99 to 11.10 mmol/L), but it may appear in the urine at different serum glucose levels, varying in individuals. Glucosuria should be distinguished from other sugars in the urine, such as lactosuria and galactosuria. In addition to the blood glucose level, other factors that affect the appearance of glucose in the urine include glomerular blood flow, tubular reabsorption rate, and urine flow. Follow-up studies are necessary to discover whether the glucosuria is caused by hyperglycemia or renal tubular dysfunction.[1,2]

1. In patients with glucosuria, assess the clinical findings, request a complete urinalysis including microscopic examination of the urinary sediment, and measure serum glucose, creatinine, and urea nitrogen.

Glucosuria may occur as an isolated finding on urinalysis, or it may be accompanied by other abnormal findings. A complete urinalysis can provide clues to a variety of disorders, such as diabetic nephropathy and urinary tract infection. A serum glucose measurement can help determine whether glucosuria is an overflow phenomenon or related to a renal disorder, and serum urea nitrogen and creatinine measurements are useful to assess renal function.

2. Evaluate the tests.

Urinary glucose can be measured by reduction methods (the usual copper reduction test) or enzymatic methods (dipstick test using glucose oxidase). Reduction methods are not specific for glucose, and a positive urinary test using a reduction method must be confirmed by an enzymatic method. Large doses of ascorbic acid (vitamin C) can cause a false-negative urinary glucose test using the glucose oxidase method. Ascorbic acid does not affect reduction methods, but other drugs can give false-positive or unusual colors with the Clinitest copper reduction test, especially the cephalosporins (Keflex) and radiocontrast agents. If urinary glucose measures positive using a reduction method and negative using glucose oxidase, tests for other urinary sugars, such as lactose and galactose, are necessary.[3,IV]

3.   If the serum glucose level is elevated in a patient with glucosuria, conclude that the urinary glucose is an overflow phenomenon, and determine whether the elevated serum glucose is from diabetes mellitus or some other cause for hyperglycemia.

Serum glucose may be increased in diabetes mellitus, in stress, and in a variety of diseases and disorders such as pancreatitis, central nervous system lesions, and secondary to drugs, for example, corticosteroids.

4.   If the serum glucose level is normal in a patient with glucosuria, consider renal tubular dysfunction.

Glucosuria without hyperglycemia is usually caused by renal tubular dysfunction, which may be inherited (uncommon) or acquired. In renal tubular dysfunction glucose is not the only substance with impaired tubular reabsorption. For example, in Fanconi's syndrome, the reabsorption of water, amino acids, sodium, bicarbonate, and phosphate is also impaired. Other examples of conditions associated with tubular dysfunction include galactosemia, cystinosis, lead poisoning, and myeloma.

REFERENCES

1.   Freeman JA, Beeler MF: Laboratory Medicine/Urinalysis and Medical Microscopy, 2nd ed. Philadelphia, Lea & Febiger, 1983.
2.   Kiel DP, Moskowitz MA: The urinalysis: A critical appraisal. Med Clin North Am 71:607, 1987.
3.   Pesce AJ, Kaplan LA: Methods in Clinical Chemistry. St Louis, The CV Mosby Co, 1987, pp 412, 1005.

PROTEINURIA

Proteinuria is a common and easily detected sign of renal disease. In the past, normal urine was thought to be free of protein. Now we know that healthy individuals excrete a small amount of protein, which is undetectable by routine methods. Normally, the composition of urinary protein is about 40% albumin, 40% tissue proteins from renal and other urogenital tissues, 15% immunoglobulins, and 5% other plasma proteins. Proteinuria may be caused by (1) an overflow of elevated plasma proteins, (2) increased glomerular permeability, (3) tubular proteinuria, and (4) altered renal hemodynamics. The presence of excessive protein indicates renal dysfunction, but whether there is significant renal disease depends on the nature, amount, and clinical setting of proteinuria. Proteinuria may be characterized as transient, orthostatic or postural, and persistent. The diagnosis depends on studying urinary and plasma proteins in the context of clinical findings, radiographs, and other laboratory studies (including renal biopsy) to document the nature and cause of the proteinuria. Clinical findings are those of the underlying disorders, for example, multiple myeloma, glomerulonephritis, interstitial nephritis, or congestive heart failure.[5,6]

1. In patients with proteinuria, assess the clinical findings, request a complete urinalysis including microscopic examination of the urinary sediment, and measure serum creatinine and urea nitrogen. Consider testing diabetics for microalbuminuria with a special method.

Proteinuria may occur as an isolated finding on urinalysis or together with other abnormal findings. A urinalysis can provide clues to a variety of disorders, such as fatty casts, oval fat bodies, and doubly refractile fat globules for the nephrotic syndrome; red cell casts for glomerulonephritis; and glucosuria for diabetes mellitus. When these other findings are present, they corroborate the significance of the proteinuria. Serum creatinine and urea nitrogen measurements are useful to evaluate renal function.

Many diabetologists believe that the early detection and reversal of microalbuminuria in diabetics may delay or prevent frank diabetic nephropathy. The usual dipstick is not sensitive enough to screen for microalbuminuria.[4]

Digital rectal examination of the prostate does not cause proteinuria.[3]

2. Evaluate the tests.

Urinary protein can be measured by dipstick, turbidimetric, chemical, and immunologic methods. With dipstick methods, false-positive results can occur with highly concentrated urine; highly alkaline (pH > 7) urine; and contamination of the urine with bacteria, blood, quaternary ammonium compounds, and chlorhexidine. False-negative results can occur with urinary immunoglobulin light chains (Bence Jones protein) and highly dilute urine. With turbidimetric methods, false-positive results can occur if the urine contains tolbutamide, radiocontrast agents, or high levels of cephalosporin, penicillin, or sulfonamide derivatives.

The usual dipstick can detect 100 to 250 mg/L of protein and is less sensitive to globulin, Bence Jones protein, or mucoprotein. To quantify microalbuminuria, a special method is necessary: a detection limit of at least 5 mg/L and a range of 5 to 200 mg/L are preferred; normal levels are below 20 mg/L. Available methods include radioimmunoassay, radial immunodiffusion, enzyme-linked immunosorbent assay (ELISA), and immunoturbidimetric technique. A tablet screening technique appears to lack sensitivity. A latex agglutination inhibition technique may prove more reliable but must be confirmed. The collection method must be standardized.[4,5]

3. If proteinuria is truly positive, measure serum creatinine, urea nitrogen, and a 24-hour protein excretion (alternatively, measure urinary protein and creatinine in a random urine specimen and calculate the protein/creatinine ratio to quantify protein excretion).* Consider the possibility of transient and orthostatic proteinuria.

Transient proteinuria may be associated with strenuous exercise, emotional stress, extreme cold, epinephrine administration, congestive heart failure, and seizures. Transient proteinuria can be documented by additional protein-free urinalyses after the precipitating cause has passed. The mechanism of proteinuria is believed to be related to hemodynamic changes. The patient should be reassured, and no further workup is indicated.

Orthostatic proteinuria is characterized by the presence of proteinuria in the erect position and absence of proteinuria (dipstick negative or <50 mg/L) in the recumbent position. The true mechanism is unknown but is believed to be increased glomerular permeability. The proteinuria usually does not exceed 2 g/day. Long-term follow-up studies over several decades have shown excellent prognosis with normal renal function.[6]

4. If proteinuria is persistent and nonorthostatic, perform a more extensive evaluation. Other useful laboratory tests include complement studies, serum albumin, serum total protein, serum and urinary immunoelectrophoresis, and radiologic evaluation.[6]

The spectrum of lesions in isolated proteinuria is wide. In patients with fixed proteinuria of less than 2 g/day without hematuria, systemic disease, or impaired renal function, renal biopsy is usually not performed unless a change in clinical status occurs or the patient requests a biopsy for other purposes. Nephrotoxic agents, such as gold salts and nonsteroidal antiinflammatory drugs, are an important cause of proteinuria that should be considered.

REFERENCES

1. Boler L, Zbella EA, Gleicher N: Quantitation of proteinuria in pregnancy by the use of single voided urine samples. Obstet Gynecol 70:99, 1987.
2. Faulkner WR: Assessment of proteinuria. Lab Report for Physicians 9:92, 1987.
3. Fincher RE, Kuske TT, Richards JW: Is digital rectal examination in men a cause of transient proteinuria? Am J Med 84:791, 1988.
4. Hindmarsh JT: Microalbuminuria. Clin Lab Med 8:611, 1988.
5. Kiel DP, Moskowitz MA: The urinalysis: A critical appraisal. Med Clin North Am 71:607, 1987.
6. Kim MS: Proteinuria. Clin Lab Med 8:527, 1988.
7. Schwab SJ, Christensen RL, Dougherty K, et al: Quantitation of proteinuria by the use of protein-to-creatinine ratios in single urine samples. Arch Intern Med 147:943, 1987.

---

*Spot urine measurements of protein and creatinine have been shown to reliably detect significant proteinuria. This avoids the cumbersome, inconvenient, and often unreliable collection of a 24-hour urine sample. Protein/creatinine ratios can distinguish healthy individuals from those with renal disease and can differentiate nephrotic range proteinuria from that seen in other renal diseases. Protein/creatinine ratios in healthy subjects seldom exceed 100 mg/g. For patients with nephrotic range proteinuria (>4.0 g/day), the ratio exceeds 2000 mg/g.[1,2,7]

HEMATURIA AND COLORED URINE*

Hematuria may be either gross (red, red-brown, or brown-black urine) or microscopic (greater than two erythrocytes per high-power field). It may be caused by a disorder of hemostasis, or it may originate in a lesion located anywhere in the urinary tract. When hematuria is gross, it is important to determine that the color of the urine is really caused by blood and not another colored substance, such as myoglobin or porphyrins. The diagnosis of the cause of hematuria depends on clinical findings, radiographs, urologic procedures, and laboratory tests. It is helpful to know whether the hematuria is painful or painless and whether it is accompanied by other urinary abnormalities, such as protein and formed elements in the urine.[3,4,8]

1. In patients with hematuria or colored urine, assess the clinical findings, request a complete urinalysis, and measure serum creatinine, urea nitrogen, creatine kinase, and haptoglobin. Obtain a carefully drawn serum specimen for visual inspection.

In hemoglobinuria, erythrocytes may be present or absent in the urinary sediment. If erythrocytes are absent and the urinary dipstick test for blood is positive, hemoglobinuria must be distinguished from myoglobinuria. If a carefully drawn serum specimen can be examined (avoiding hemolysis), it will often be pink with hemoglobinemia but a normal color with myoglobinemia, because serum myoglobin is rapidly cleared by the kidneys but serum hemoglobin is not. Additional useful tests are a serum creatine kinase (CK), which will often be markedly increased in myoglobinuria secondary to muscle damage, and serum haptoglobin, which will be low in hemoglobinuria and normal in myoglobinuria.

Hematuria may be present as an isolated finding on urinalysis or together with other abnormal findings. A complete urinalysis can provide clues to a variety of disorders such as urinary tract infection and urinary calculi. Creatinine and urea nitrogen measurements are useful to assess renal function.

2. Evaluate the tests.

The usual dipstick test relies on the peroxidase-like activity of erythrocytes and hemoglobin. Both hemoglobin and myoglobin give a positive test result. False-positive results may occur when testing urine from menstruating women or when the urine is contaminated with residues of strongly oxidizing cleaning agents in the urine container or with povidone-iodine. False-negative readings may occur when the urine contains large quantities of ascorbic acid (vitamin C) or when the urine is preserved with formalin.[8]

Currently available dipsticks are capable of detecting two or three erythrocytes per high-power field with a sensitivity of 97%. Intact erythrocytes hemolyze on the dipstick, and the liberated hemoglobin produces a colored dot. Scattered or compacted dots indicate intact erythrocytes, whereas a uniform green color indicates free hemoglobin, hemolyzed erthrocytes, or myoglobin.[8]

---

*Includes discussion of hemoglobinuria, myoglobinuria, and other pigments.

3. In patients with documented gross or microscopic hematuria, determine the source of the hemoglobin or bleeding.

Hemoglobinuria can be caused by hemolytic disorders, which may be either inherited or acquired. After a race, marathon runners may have hematuria. Myoglobinuria can be caused by rhabdomyolsis, which may occur in the following conditions: primary muscle injury, increased muscle energy consumption (strenuous exercise, status epilepticus), decreased muscle energy consumption (diabetic ketoacidosis), decreased muscle oxygenation, infections, and toxins.[9]

The most common causes of hematuria originating in the urinary tract are cystitis, urethritis, and bleeding from the prostate; the most serious are bladder and kidney carcinoma, urinary calculi, and renal tuberculosis. Glomerulonephritis is an important cause of hematuria, in which the question of whether or not to perform a renal biopsy is often raised. About 10% of patients with gross hematuria and 35% with microscopic hematuria have so-called essential hematuria of unknown cause.[3,5,6,10]

Cytologic examination of the urine without endoscopic examination of the bladder may be a simple, cost-effective method for evaluating asymptomatic microhematuria in women.[1] In patients with idiopathic hematuria, renal biopsy makes no difference therapeutically or probably prognostically; and therefore it should not be considered necessary for routine management of asymptomatic hematuria.[5]

If no pathologic cause for hematuria is present, consider an entity known as familial hematuria in which hematuria is present in other family members and good renal function is maintained during long follow-up.[2]

4. In patients with red or brown urine, if the dipstick test for blood is negative, conclude that a substance other than hemoglobin or myoglobin is responsible for the colored urine.

Red, red-brown, or brown-black urine may result from either ingested substances or substances that originate in the body. Ingested substances include azodyes (pyridium), phenolsulfonphthalein, para-aminosalicylic acid, anthraquinones, nitrofurantoin, metronidazole, sulfa compounds, chloroquine, methyldopa, levodopa, phenacetin, salicylates, methocarbamol, cresol, iron sorbitol citrate, and beets (individuals who can absorb betanin). Phenytoin is not a cause of red urine.[7] Substances originating in the body include bilirubin, porphyrin, melanin (in melanoma), homogentisic acid (in alkaptonuria), and the red pigment produced by *Serratia marcescens* (in infection by that organism).[9]

5. In patients with myoglobinuria (acute rhabdomyolysis), the following additional abnormal laboratory test results may occur[9]:

CHEMISTRY

• Serum urea nitrogen/creatinine ratio is frequently decreased ($<$10:1), because creatine from injured muscles is rapidly converted into creatinine.
• Elevated uric acid caused by conversion of muscle purines to uric acid. Renal failure may further elevate uric acid.

- Depressed calcium (early) followed by elevated calcium (later). Possible deposition of calcium in damaged muscle tissue.
- Elevated phosphate probably from muscle. Renal failure may further elevate phosphate.
- Hyperkalemia from muscle.

REFERENCES

1. Bard RH: The significance of asymptomatic microhematuria in women and its economic implications. Arch Intern Med 148:2629, 1988.
2. Benign familial hematuria. Lancet 2:549, 1988.
3. Bloom KJ: An algorithm for hematuria. Clin Lab Med 8:577, 1988.
4. Connelly J, Griner PF: Microscopic hematuria. In Griner PF, Panzer RJ, Greenland P: Clinical Diagnosis and the Laboratory: Logical Strategies for Common Medical Problems. Chicago, Year Book Medical Publishers, Inc, 1986, p 366.
5. Copley JB, Hasbargen JA: "Idiopathic" hematuria: A prospective evaluation. Arch Intern Med 147:434, 1987.
6. Corwin HL, Silverstein MD: Microscopic hematuria. Clin Lab Med 8:601, 1988.
7. Derby BM, Ward JW: The myth of red urine due to phenytoin. JAMA 249:1723, 1983.
8. Kiel DP, Moskowitz MA: The urinalysis: A critical appraisal. Med Clin North Am 71:607, 1987.
9. Materson BJ, Preston RA: Myoglobinuria versus hemoglobinuria. Hospital Practice, October 30, 1988, p 29.
10. Thompson IM: The evaluation of microscopic hematuria: A population-based study. J Urol 138:1189, 1987.

COMMUNITY-ACQUIRED URINARY TRACT INFECTION IN WOMEN

Of all infections, urinary tract infection (UTI) is one of the most common. Except in male neonates with urogenital anatomic abnormalities and men over 50 years old with prostatic hypertrophy and obstruction, UTI is predominantly a disease of women. UTI is common in women of all ages with a prevalence of 1% to 2% by 20 years of age and an increase of 1% per decade of life thereafter. Most of these women with UTI have normal urinary anatomy. Because a short urethra may predispose to UTI, proper cleansing after a bowel movement and frequent and complete urination (including urination after sexual intercourse) are important measures to prevent UTIs in women. UTI may involve the upper urinary tract, such as the kidneys, or the lower urinary tract, such as the bladder and urethra. Over 95% of UTIs are caused by a single bacterial species, and over 90% of these species are Gram-negative bacilli or enterococci. The infection may be superficial, as in the mucosa of the bladder, or deep, as in the kidneys. Along with clinical findings and radiographic studies, laboratory tests play an important role in diagnosis. Patients with UTI may be asymptomatic with bacteriuria, have findings of cystitis, have a full-blown pyelonephritis, or have the acute urethral syndrome with few to no urinary bacteria, for example, dysuria caused by *Neisseria gonorrhoeae* or *Chlamydia trachomatis*. This discussion will be limited to community-acquired UTI in women.[2,3,6,7]

1. **In women with clinical findings of a lower UTI, request a urinalysis. If the clinical findings suggest pyelonephritis (fever, rigors, nausea, vomiting, flank pain, costovertebral angle tenderness), obtain a urine Gram stain and a urine culture.***

Patients with findings of lower UTI and possible subclinical pyelonephritis (pregnancy, underlying urinary tract disease, diabetes mellitus, immunosuppression, symptoms for more than 7 days, three or more UTIs in past year, past history of pyelonephritis, recent use of antibiotics, poor city neighborhood) should have a urine Gram stain and culture as well as a urinalysis.[4,8,9]

For sexually active patients with possible chlamydial or gonococcal urethritis, request a urinalysis and obtain a Gram stain and culture of urethral (or cervical os) discharge.† Urethritis in the sexual partner, a new sexual partner, or mucopurulent endocervical secretions are suggestive.[4]

For women with findings of vaginitis, obtain a microscopic examination of any abnormal vaginal discharge.‡

Since the decision to treat a lower UTI is based on the presence of pyuria rather than bacteriuria, only a urinalysis is required when the clinical findings are limited to the lower urinary tract, for example, dysuria, urgency, and frequency.

Since false-negative results with the dipstick nitrite test may occur when the urine has not been retained in the bladder long enough for Gram-negative bacteria to reduce nitrates in the urine to nitrites, a first-morning urine specimen is best. Other causes of a false-negative nitrite test are deficient dietary nitrate and urinary ascorbic acid concentration of 75 mg/dl (4.28 mmol/L) or greater.[6] Other factors that can influence test results include hydration status (is patient forcing fluids?), urinary pH, antibiotics, and other drugs.

---

*Women should be requested to manually clean the labia and area around the urethral meatus thoroughly with a mild soap and water solution, again stroking away from the meatus of the urethra once it has been cleaned. In a squatting position, either over a bedpan or on a toilet seat, the female patient should be told to separate the labia with one hand and begin voiding. During the void, preferably at the approximate midpoint, a collection bottle or cup held in the other hand should be inserted into the urine stream without the void being halted. When an adequate sample has been collected, the cup should be withdrawn and the patient instructed to complete the urination into the toilet or bedpan.[5]

†Specimens for gonococcal culture should include cervical and rectal swabs, and the urethra may also be sampled. Maximal recovery of *Chlamydia* is achieved by culture of both cervix and urethra. These specimens should be collected with synthetic fiber swabs, because wooden shafts and calcium alginate swabs are toxic to chlamydia and to a lesser extent to gonococci. Chlamydia cultures require immediate inoculation of the specimen into a suitable transport medium, such as 2SP. Cultures for gonococci taken in a physician's office should be immediately cultured and placed in an incubator at 35°C in 5% to 10% CO_2, and these cultures should be incubated overnight before being sent to a laboratory for analysis.

‡Microscopic examination using a drop of 10% KOH to dissolve cellular material is useful to identify the pseudohyphae and budding forms of *Candida;* a Gram stain is also helpful. A wet mount of fresh discharge with a drop of warm normal saline can be prepared to identify the motile flagellated *Trichomonas* and "clue" cells, which are bacilli within epithelial cells that are often present in patients with *Gardnerella vaginitis* (formerly *Haemophilus vaginitis*). Cultures are necessary to diagnose the rare cases of purulent vaginitis from gonorrhea.

After collection, the urine specimen should be promptly (within 20 minutes) cultured or refrigerated if culture is delayed.[8] A Gram stain of mixed but unspun urine is a rapid test for the presence of leukocytes and bacteria over 100,000/ml that may be useful in the office or clinic setting.

2. Evaluate the tests.

ORGANISM	APPROXIMATE PERCENTAGE OF PATIENTS
Escherichia coli	85–90%
Enterococci	2–5%
*Staphylococcus saprophyticus**	2–4%
Other Gram-negative bacteria	1–9%

*Significant pathogen in young, sexually active women.

Whenever mixed bacterial species are grown on culture, the likelihood of contamination is high. Moreover, *Staphylococcus epidermidis,* diphtheroids, and lactobacilli are commonly found in the distal urethra and rarely cause infection. If contamination is suspected and culture results are still important, the culture should be repeated.[V]

3.   Interpret pyuria, Gram stains, and urine cultures in the context of the clinical findings.

LOWER URINARY TRACT INFECTION

In patients with findings of lower UTI the presence of pyuria justifies giving immediate therapy, whereas the absence of pyuria justifies withholding therapy. Pyuria is present in 90% to 95% of patients with lower UTI and colony counts over 100,000 bacteria/ml of urine, in 70% of patients with lower UTI and colony counts of 100 to 100,000 bacteria/ml, and in only 1% of asymptomatic nonbacteriuric patients. It the patient has pyuria without bacteriuria (by examination of unstained sediment), consider chlamydial urethritis, gonococcal urethritis, or urinary infection with Gram-positive cocci. Lower UTI caused by yeasts (*Candida* species, *Torulopsis*) may also exhibit pyuria. Urinary tract yeast infections are important and are more common in diabetics.[1,8,10]

PYELONEPHRITIS

In patients with findings of acute pyelonephritis or subclinical pyelonephritis, urinalysis typically shows pyuria with possible proteinuria, hematuria, and casts. A urine Gram stain and culture are necessary to isolate the responsible organism and identify the pattern of antibacterial sensitivities. Usually, but not always, the colony count will be greater than 100,000 bacteria/ml of urine.[1,8]

CHLAMYDIAL URETHRITIS

Urethral infection with *Chlamydia trachomatis* accounts for 2% to 20% of cases of acute dysuria in women. The urinalysis shows pyuria without bacteriuria.

Hematuria is very unusual, as is proteinuria. Routine urine culture will not isolate *C. trachomatis* and will often be negative for other organisms. Recently developed rapid assays for chlamydial antigens using monoclonal antibodies appear highly sensitive and specific. The sensitivity of a single culture for *Chlamydia* is about 80%. The sensitivity of nonculture, rapid antigen detection systems is about 60% to 90% when compared to culture, and the sensitivity is highly dependent on the skill of the technologist. Although some reagents are highly specific, others are less specific, so that some false-positive results may be obtained with rapid assays.[2,4,8]

GONOCOCCAL URETHRITIS

Neisseria gonorrhoeae typically produces pyuria. Gram stain shows Gram-negative intracellular diplococci, and culture on Thayer-Martin or New York City medium will isolate the organism. Positive Gram stains of cervical discharge are suggestive but not diagnostic of gonococci. These Gram stains should be interpreted with caution if vaginal epithelial cells are present, because anaerobic Gram-negative bacteria and coccobacillary bacteria may resemble gonococci.[1,8]

OTHER URETHRAL INFECTIONS

Urethritis may also be caused by herpes simplex, *Trichomonas vaginalis,* and *Candida albicans.* Herpes simplex and *Trichomonas vaginalis* produce pyuria, but candidal infection does not.[4,8]

VAGINITIS

Patients with vaginitis may have dysuria (plus frequency and urgency) as their chief complaint. Typically pyuria is absent, except when trichomonal infection involves the urethra as well as the vagina. Microscopic examination of the abnormal discharge may reveal budding yeast and pseudohyphae, trichomonads, and "clue cells."[1,8]

ASYMPTOMATIC WOMEN WITH BACTERIURIA

The value of identifying asymptomatic bacteriuria (>100,000 bacteria/ml) in asymptomatic, nonpregnant women is controversial. Asymptomatic bacteriuria appears to be correlated with increased mortality in the elderly, but there is no evidence that treatment alters the mortality. *It is important to treat asymptomatic bacteriuria in pregnant women, since therapy reduces the occurrence of acute pyelonephritis and possibly low-birth-weight babies. Therefore pregnant women should have regular urinalyses in the prenatal period with urine cultures if pyuria is noted.*[1,8]

SYMPTOMATIC WOMEN WITHOUT PYURIA

Many women with dysuria have no pyuria, have no recognized pathogen, and do not respond to antimicrobial treatment. These women should have a urinalysis and urine culture.[9] In these women, consider urethral inflammation from physical or chemical agents of from trauma.[1,8]

REFERENCES

1. Corriere JN, Hanno PM, Hooton T, et al: Cystitis: Evolving standard of care. Patient Care, February 29, 1988, p 33.
2. Fang LST: Urinalysis in the diagnosis of urinary tract infections. Clin Lab Med 8:567, 1988.
3. Forland M: Frequent and painful urination (urinary tract infection). In Cutler P: Problem Solving in Clinical Medicine: From Data to Diagnosis, 2nd ed. Baltimore, Williams & Wilkins, 1985, p 422.
4. General Internal Medicine Subspecialty Committee: Medical Knowledge Self-Assessment Program VIII. General Internal Medicine. Philadelphia, American College of Physicians, 1988, p 8.
5. Haber MH: Quality assurance in urinalysis. Clin Lab Med 8:431, 1988.
6. Kiel DP, Moskowitz MA: The urinalysis: A critical appraisal. Med Clin North Am 71:607, 1987.
7. Komaroff AL: Acute dysuria in adult women. In Griner PF, Panzer RJ, Greenland P: Clinical Diagnosis and the Laboratory: Logical Strategies for Common Medical Problems. Chicago, Year Book Medical Publishers, Inc, 1986, p 346.
8. Komaroff AL: Urinalysis and urine culture in women with dysuria. In Sox HC (ed): Common Diagnostic Tests. Use and Interpretation. Philadelphia, American College of Physicians, 1987, p 238.
9. Sodeman TM: Urinalysis and urine culture in women with dysuria. In Glenn GC (ed): Blue Cross/Blue Shield Association Guidelines Based on Common Diagnostic Tests. Use and Interpretation. Skokie, IL, College of American Pathologists, 1988, p 15.
10. Urinary tract candidosis. Lancet 2:1000, 1988.

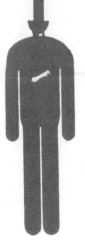

CHAPTER 8

ENDOCRINE AND METABOLIC DISORDERS

HYPERTHYROIDISM AND HYPOTHYROIDISM

Thyroid disorders are among the most frequently encountered endocrinologic problems, and the use of laboratory tests is essential to the diagnosis of both the hyperthyroid and the hypothyroid state. The strategy for differentiating hyperthyroidism and hypothyroidism from euthyroidism centers on the measurement of serum thyroxine; however, thyroxine can be falsely elevated or depressed secondary to changes in thyroid-binding globulin (TBG). Actually, the serum active hormone is free thyroxine, and because free thyroxine is not easily measured, certain indirect tests, such as the free thyroxine index, which is the product of the serum thyroxine and the triiodothyronine resin uptake, have emerged. Although thyroxine is the major secretory product of the thyroid gland, triiodothyronine is the major metabolically active hormone. About 80% of triiodothyronine is generated outside the thyroid, principally in the liver and kidney, by removal of the iodine atom in the 5' position of the outer ring of thyroxine. If the inner-ring iodine in the 5' position is removed, the metabolically inactive, reverse triiodothyronine is formed. In contrast to the old thyrotropin (thyroid-stimulating hormone) test, which can only detect hypothyroidism, a new highly sensitive thyrotropin test (S-TSH) has recently been developed, which is capable of detecting hyperthyroidism as well as hypothyroidism. The increasing complexity of thyroid tests and confusion in nomenclature have recently been addressed by the American Thyroid Association.[1,3,4,7,10]

1. In patients with clinical findings of either hyperthyroidism or hypothyroidism or if you wish to screen for these disorders, request a total serum thyroxine (T₄), a triiodothyronine resin uptake (T₃RU), and a calculated free thyroxine index (FT₄I). Alternatively, consider requesting the new highly sensitive thyrotropin test (S-TSH), a test that is probably superior to other tests and that may even replace them.*

To increase the sensitivity of the testing strategy, and to save time, in patients with findings of hyperthyroidism, initially request a triiodothyronine (T₃) test together with the T₄, T₃RU, and FT₄I tests, and in patients with findings of hypothyroidism, initially request a TSH test together with the T₄, T₃RU, and FT₄I tests. Screening for thyroid disease is not productive except perhaps in patients with hypercholesterolemia or for thyroid dysfunction in elderly patients with cardiac disease such as worsening angina, unexplained congestive heart failure,

---

*As more experience is gained with the new S-TSH and as it becomes more standardized , it may become the single most cost-effective screening test for thyroid disease currently available.[5] At present, the cost of the S-TSH tends to be higher than older thyroid function tests.[7]

113

or atrial fibrillation. Periodic testing to detect hyperthyroidism in the elderly is appropriate, because thyroid dysfunction is more prevalent and symptoms are unreliable.[8] *It is better not to request routine thyroid function tests in seriously ill patients, since falsely abnormal results may occur (euthyroid sick syndrome).*

One may initially order only a serum T_4 to evaluate hyperthyroidism or hypothyroidism and depend on clinical information to alert one to situations where serum TBG is increased or decreased, causing false-positive or false-negative T_4 results. Because these situations may be difficult to recognize, a better approach is to initially order a T_3RU and a calculated FT_4 I together with the T_4 or order an S-TSH.

Clinical situations in which the concentration of TBG and T_4 may be increased include newborns; porphyria; cirrhosis; acute hepatitis; pregnancy; oral contraceptive administration; therapy with estrogens, opiates, perphenazine, and clofibrate; in certain families; and after administration of heroin or methadone. In these situations, the increased T_4 would be falsely positive for hyperthyroidism. TBG and T_4 may be decreased in chronic protein malnutrition; hepatic failure; nephrotic syndrome; chronic illness; in certain families; and after administration of L-asparaginase, androgenic steroids, or glucocorticoids. In these situations, the decreased T_4 would be falsely positive for hypothyroidism.

If your laboratory offers the new highly sensitive test for serum thyrotropin (S-TSH), you may use it instead of the T_4, T_3RU, and FT_4I. The new S-TSH test can detect hyperthyroidism (low TSH) or hypothyroidism (high TSH). The old TSH test was not sensitive enough to detect the low levels of TSH found in hyperthyroidism and was only good to detect the high levels of TSH seen in hypothyroidism. You may also use the direct measurement of free thyroxine (FT_4) instead of the T_4, T_3RU, and FT_4I; however, the FT_4 is not widely available.

2. If the diagnosis of hypothyroidism is in doubt and the patient is taking thyroid hormone replacement, discontinue thyroid medication and after 5 weeks measure the serum T_4, T_3RU, FT_4I, and serum TSH.

After 5 weeks without thyroid medication, an elevated TSH reliably separates patients with hypothyroidism from patients who are euthyroid (normal TSH). Of course, therapy must be resumed if the patient is hypothyroid.[v]

3. Evaluate the tests. See table on p. 115.

4. If the serum FT_4I is increased, the diagnosis is probably hyperthyroidism, but remember that some euthyroid patients may have increased serum FT_4I values. Obtain an S-TSH in doubtful cases.

The S-TSH level is depressed in hypothyroidism; however, exceptions have been noted. In a group composed of both inpatients and outpatients with suppressed thyrotropin levels, 17% had this finding from causes other than thyrotoxicosis, including central hypothyroidism, acute psychiatric illness, and medications. This finding was prevalent in hospitalized patients in whom nonthyroidal illness, or drug therapy (especially glucocorticoids and dopamine) or both, cause suppression of thyrotropin even when thyroxine levels are normal or low.[5,7]

REFERENCE RANGE VALUES[x]

TEST	SPECIMEN	REFERENCE RANGE (CONVENTIONAL)	REFERENCE RANGE (INTERNATIONAL)
Free Thyroxine index (FT$_4$I)	Serum	1.2–5.0	1.2–5.0

Thyroxine (T$_4$), total	Serum	10–60 yr: 5–12 μg/dl
		>60 yr
		  M*: 5–10 μg/dl
		  F†: 5.5–10.5 μg/dl
			65–155 nmol/L
			
			65–129 nmol/L
			71–135 nmol/L

Triiodothyronine resin uptake test (T$_3$RU)	Serum	Adult: 24–34%	24–34 AU‡

Triiodothyronine (T$_3$), total	Serum	120–195 ng/dl
		>60 yr
		  M: 105–175 ng/dl
		  F: 108–205 ng/dl
			1.85–3.00 nmol/L
			
			1.62–2.69 nmol/L
			1.66–3.16 nmol/L

Thyroxine, free (FT$_4$)	Serum	0.8–2.4 ng/dl	10–31 pmol/L
Thyrotropin (thyroid-stimulating hormone; TSH)	Serum	<10 μIU/ml	<10 mIU/L
Thyrotropin (S-TSH)§[7]	Serum	0.4–6.0 μIU/ml	0.4–6.0 mIU/L

*Male.
† Female.
‡ Arbitrary units.
§ Subclinical hypothyroidism has been recognized for 20 yr and is characterized by patients who are clinically euthyroid and have normal or equivocal serum T$_4$ and T$_3$ concentrations and an increased TSH. With the new S-TSH a group of patients will be recognized who have subclinical hyperthyroidism (i.e., clinically euthyroid, normal or equivocal serum T$_4$ and T$_3$ concentrations, and decreased S-TSH level).[7]

Almost all hyperthyroid patients will have an increased FT$_4$I and T$_3$ (also an increased free T$_3$ and free T$_3$ index [FT$_3$I]). Since the concentration of T$_3$ varies with TBGs, it may be useful to calculate the FT$_3$I. About 5% of hyperthyroid patients will have a normal FT$_4$I and an increased T$_3$ and FT$_3$I.

An increased FT$_4$I can occur in severe nonthyroid illness, such as hyperemesis gravidarum. The mechanism for the increased T$_4$ is thought to be impaired conversion of T$_4$ to triiodothyronine (T$_3$). Along with the fall in T$_3$ levels there is a rise in reverse T$_3$ levels (rT$_3$). Other euthyroid patients may have an increased serum T$_4$ when taking certain drugs, such as amiodarone, iopanoic acid, ipodate, propylthiouracil, propranolol, and glucocorticoids, which impair the conversion of T$_4$ to T$_3$. The FT$_4$I values are usually normal in these circumstances but may be high with amiodarone. Still other euthyroid patients may have familial abnormalities that cause an increased T_4 or FT_4I. The clue to false-positive elevations of FT_4I are a normal T_3 and a normal FT_3I.

5. If the serum FT₄I is normal, the patient is probably euthyroid. Remember that about 5% of hyperthyroid patients and an even larger number of hypothyroid patients may have a normal FT₄I (request a T₃ or TSH). Alternatively, obtain an S-TSH in doubtful cases.

The S-TSH level is normal in euthyroidism; however, exceptions have been noted. The serum thyrotropin level is normal in untreated central hypothyroidism. Similarly, thyrotropin may be normal or elevated in states of generalized resistance to thyroid hormone and thyrotoxicosis induced by thyrotropin-producing tumors.[5,7] In hyperthyroidism with a normal FT_4I, the T_3 is usually elevated, and in hypothyroidism with a normal FT_4I, the TSH is usually elevated.

6. If the serum FT₄I is normal, low, or borderline-low and the diagnosis of hypothyroidism is suspected, order a TSH. Remember that some euthyroid patients with severe nonthyroid illness may have a low FT₄I.

The S-TSH level is elevated in hypothyroidism; however, exceptions have been noted. Elevated thyrotropin levels are common in patients hospitalized with psychiatric illness: the FT_4I may be normal or elevated. After 1 or more weeks the serum thyrotropin and thyroxine levels return to normal in most patients.[5,7]

In many hypothyroid patients the T_4, FT_4I, and T_3 may be normal or borderline-low and an increased TSH is required to support the diagnosis. This is because an increased TSH is the most sensitive test for primary hypothyroidism. Subclinical hypothyroidism refers to patients who are clinically euthyroid but who have an increased TSH level and a normal or an equivocal FT_4I level. Almost all patients with symptomatic hypothyroidism will have TSH levels greater than 20 mIU/ml and those with minimal findings will have levels between 10 and 20 mIU/ml. An increase in TSH establishes the diagnosis of primary hypothyroidism.

TSH values are not always elevated in hypothyroidism. Since administration of thyroid-releasing hormone (TRH) stimulates a greater elevation of TSH in hypothyroid than in normal or hyperthyroid patients, the TRH stimulation test may be useful in doubtful cases of hypothyroidism.

In patients with hypothalamic or pituitary hypothyroidism (central or secondary hypothyroidism) the TSH may not be elevated and other hormones such as serum gonadotropin, prolactin, and cortisol should be measured to document pituitary failure. Hypothalamic or pituitary causes account for less than 10% of hypothyroid cases.

Patients with severe nonthyroid illness may have false-positive tests for hypothyroidism, that is, low FT_4I.

7. If you conclude that the diagnosis is hypothyroidism and decide to treat the patient with thyroxine, dessicated thyroid, or triiodothyronine, measure the serum TSH level (preferably using the S-TSH) to monitor therapy.

Until the TSH level is normal, full replacement therapy has not been achieved. Patients on replacement therapy should be observed for clinical features of excess hormone and the thyrotropin level should be measured to detect inadequate replacement. Serum T_4 and T_3 are not reliable guides to therapy. Excessive replacement therapy can cause osteoporosis, and the old TSH test is not sensitive enough to detect the low levels of thyrotropin found in hyperthyroidism. Consider using the S-TSH to monitor therapy, since it can detect overtreatment as well as undertreatment. The ideal dose of thyroid hormone will lower the S-TSH level into the normal but not the subnormal range. The patient should have received a given dose of hormone for about 6 weeks before measuring thyrotropin and considering a change in dosage.[2,5,6,7] T_4 and FT_4I measurements are not needed if the TSH level is normal, but they should be done in patients with low TSH levels.[9]

8. If you are treating the patient with thyroid hormone to suppress TSH secretion, as in treatment of thyroid carcinoma, use the S-TSH to monitor TSH levels.

The S-TSH can distinguish suppressed levels of TSH from normal TSH levels.[5,7]

9. If you are treating patients for thyrotoxicosis or subacute thyroiditis, measuring the thyrotropin level (S-TSH) alone may not accurately reflect the patient's clinical status.

Patients recovering from or receiving antithyroid drug therapy for thyrotoxicosis and patients in the recovery phase of subacute thyroiditis when previously excessive thyroid hormone doses are reduced may have a suppressed thyrotropin level (S-TSH) even when thyroid levels are normal or low.[5]

10. In the hyperthyroid patient, the following additional abnormal laboratory test results may occur:

HEMATOLOGY

- Mild anemia of chronic disease
- Moderate neutropenia
- Elevated erythrocyte sedimentation rate (ESR)

CHEMISTRY

- Decreased PO_2
- Decreased PCO_2 with respiratory alkalosis
- Hyperglycemia from accelerated hepatic glycogenolysis secondary to increased catecholamines
- Elevated urea nitrogen and creatinine
- Hypokalemia and periodic paralysis
- Hypercalcemia caused by bone dissolution by osteoclasts
- Hypomagnesemia
- Slightly elevated aspartate aminotransferase (AST or SGOT)
- Elevated alkaline phosphatase from stimulation of osteoclasts by thyroid hormones[2]

- Hyperamylasemia in thyrotoxicosis
- Hypoalbuminemia
- Hyperbilirubinemia caused by hemolysis or hypobilirubinemia related to decreased red cell mass and hypoalbuminemia
- Hypocholesterolemia and hypotriglyceridemia
- Hypernatremia caused by hypercalcemic diabetes insipidus

11. In the hypothyroid patient, the following additional abnormal laboratory test results may occur:

HEMATOLOGY

- Mild to moderate anemia of chronic disease; sometimes pernicious anemia with Hashimoto's thyroiditis
- Elevated (ESR)

CHEMISTRY

- Depressed PO_2 with dyspnea secondary to pleural effusion
- Metabolic acidosis caused by renal insufficiency and elevated lactic acid

- Hyperglycemia and diabetes mellitus or hypoglycemia
- Slightly elevated creatinine, urea nitrogen, and uric acid, which are related to decreased glomerular filtration and which return to normal with replacement therapy; uric acid frequently elevated and may lead to attacks of gout

- Hyponatremia with or without the inappropriate ADH syndrome; may also be caused by pseudohyponatremia associated with hyperlipidemia
- Hyperkalemia caused by decreased glomerular filtration
- Hypocalcemia
- Hypermagnesemia

- Elevated creatine kinase (CK-MM variant), aspartate aminotransferase (AST or SGOT), and lactate dehydrogenase (LD) caused by skeletal muscle myopathy
- Decreased alkaline phosphatase (ALP) caused by decreased osteoblastic activity

- Hyperalbuminemia
- Hypercholesterolemia in hypothyroidism of thyroid (but not pituitary) origin[II]
- Hypertriglyceridemia
- Decreased ferritin, presumably because of retarded protein turnover

REFERENCES

1. American Thyroid Association: Revised nomenclature for tests of thyroid hormones and thyroid-related proteins in serum. J Clin Endocrinol Metab 64:1089, 1987.
2. Cooper DS: Thyroid hormone and the skeleton: A bone of contention. JAMA 259:3175, 1988.
3. Cutler P: Nervousness and weight loss (thyroid dysfunction). In Cutler P: Problem Solving in Clinical Medicine: From Data to Diagnosis, 2nd ed. Baltimore, Williams & Wilkins, 1985, p 286.

4. Dolan JG: Hyperthyroidism and hypothyroidism. In Griner PF, Panzer RJ, Greenland P: Clinical Diagnosis and the Laboratory: Logical Strategies for Common Medical Problems. Chicago, Year Book Medical Publishers, Inc, 1986, p 558.
5. Ehrmann DA, Sarne DH: Serum thyrotropin and the assessment of thyroid status. Ann Int Med 110:179, 1989.
6. Paul TL, Kerrigan JP, Kelly AM, et al: Long-term L-thyroxine therapy is associated with decreased hip bone density in premenopausal women. JAMA 259:3137, 1988.
7. Symposium on sensitive TSH assays—Introduction, Part II, Part III. Mayo Clin Proc 63:1026, 1123, 1214, 1988.
8. Tibaldi JM, Barzel US, Albin J, et al: Thyrotoxicosis in the very old. Am J Med 81:619, 1986.
9. Watts NB: Use of a sensitive thyrotropin assay for monitoring treatment with levothyroxine. Arch Intern Med 149:309, 1989.
10. Wong ET, Steffes MW: A fundamental approach to the diagnosis of diseases of the thyroid gland. Clin Lab Med 4:655, 1984.

HYPERCALCEMIA AND HYPERPARATHYROIDISM

If the Mayo Clinic experience in detecting hypercalcemia by biochemical screening is extrapolated nationwide, approximately 35,000 to 86,000 new patients with unexplained elevations of serum calcium will be discovered annually in the United States. The merits of screening for hypercalcemia are controversial. However, once discovered, patients with hypercalcemia must be studied to differentiate primary hyperparathyroidism from malignancy-associated hypercalcemia and hypercalcemia of other causes. The strategy for the differential diagnosis of hypercalcemia depends on the reliable documentation of elevated serum calcium levels in the context of a thorough workup. Cancer and primary hyperparathyroidism are common causes. Primary hyperparathyroidism is more common in patients who have had prior neck irradiation and in the elderly.[1,2,4,7,9]

1. In patients with clinical findings of hyperparathyroidism or if an individual is found to have an elevated serum calcium, request at least three measurements of serum total calcium together with a complete blood count (CBC), serum albumin and globulins by electrophoresis, phosphorus, alkaline phosphatase, urea nitrogen, creatinine, electrolytes, thyroid function tests, and a 24-hour urinary calcium. In certain circumstances, measurement of serum ionized calcium may be helpful. Check any drugs for a possible hypercalcemic effect.

These laboratory studies should be part of a thorough workup that includes a careful history and physical examination, chest roentgenography, renal ultrasonography, and skeletal survey radiographs. Drugs, such as vitamin D or antacids together with milk, can cause hypercalcemia.

In the past, patients with hyperparathyroidism were more likely to show clinical features of the disease than to show only hypercalcemia. Now, following the advent of laboratory screening, the typical presentation of patients with hyperparathyroidism is unexplained hypercalcemia. Although some experts believe that screening for hypercalcemia is valuable, others argue that there is no advantage in treating asymptomatic hyperparathyroidism and that screening for serum calcium should be omitted.

Other causes of hypercalcemia that must be differentiated from hyperparathyroidism follow:

INCREASED GASTROINTESTINAL ABSORPTION OF CALCIUM	INCREASED RESORPTION OF BONE	INCREASED RENAL RESORPTION
Sarcoidosis	Cancer of bone*	Thiazide diuretics
Other granulomatous diseases		
Milk-alkali syndrome	Ectopic PTH syndrome	Familial hypocalciuric hypercalcemia
Hypervitaminosis D	Hyperthyroidism	
	Paget's disease of bone	
	Immobilization	

*These are usually the lytic metastases of carcinoma of the breast, lung, and prostate; or multiple myeloma, acute leukemias, certain lymphomas, and Hodgkin's disease. Sometimes bone involvement is absent and the hypercalcemia is induced by a humoral mediator.

Common causes for hypercalcemia are cancer and hyperparathyroidism, and whereas most hospitalized patients with hypercalcemia will have cancer, most ambulatory patients will have hyperparathyroidism and only a few will have cancer. Other conditions associated with hypercalcemia include hypothyroidism; adrenal insufficiency; acromegaly; vitamin A intoxication; pheochromocytoma; the watery diarrhea, hypokalemia, achlorhydria syndrome; lithium therapy; and post-renal transplant patients.

Remember that posture affects serum calcium levels. Since serum calcium is bound to albumin and since albumin is higher in ambulatory than in recumbent patients, calcium is higher in ambulatory patients than in recumbent patients. Also, do not apply a tourniquet or allow muscular exercise of the limb chosen for venipuncture, since venous occlusion or muscular exercise can artifactually elevate calcium. Serum or heparinized plasma is a satisfactory sample, but do not allow prolonged contact with erythrocytes, since with time the cells become permeable to calcium. Using a cork stopper for the patient's sample can elevate the calcium level, because cork contains calcium.

Serum inorganic phosphorous concentrations are difficult to interpret unless they are collected in the morning after an overnight fast (during which there is no intravenous intake or calories). Under these conditions, the normal range for adults is 3.0 to 4.5 mg/dl (0.97 to 1.45 mmol/L). It is slightly higher before puberty and after gonadal failure.

Serum total calcium comprises three forms: a protein-bound fraction (40%); a chelated fraction (10%); and an ionized, physiologically active fraction (50%). Serum measurements of total calcium are sometimes misleading, especially among patients in intensive care units, in neonates, in patients undergoing liver and cardiac transplant surgery, and in patients with renal disease. In these patients, serum ionized calcium measurements may be helpful. Blood samples should be collected anaerobically and without venous stasis. A minimal amount of heparin and other anticoagulants should be used because they bind calcium and lower the ionized calcium level.[3,8]

2. Evaluate the tests.

REFERENCE RANGE VALUES[x]

TEST	SPECIMEN	REFERENCE RANGE (CONVENTIONAL)	REFERENCE RANGE (INTERNATIONAL)
Calcium, ionized (iCa)	Serum, plasma, or whole blood (heparin)	4.48–4.92 mg/dl	1.12–1.23 mmol/L

Make certain that serum total calcium is measured by an accurate and precise method. The reference method is atomic absorption. Using a single serum calcium measurement, the accuracy and precision of present calcium methods are not good enough to sharply distinguish normocalcemia from hypercalcemia. In addition, patients with mild hyperparathyroidism may have intermittent elevations. Therefore repeat measurements of serum calcium should be obtained.

The reference range for serum total calcium should be adjusted up or down according to the ratio of 0.8 mg/dl (0.2 mmol/L) of serum calcium for every 1 g/dl (10 g/L) of serum albumin above or below the middle of the reference range. With an increase or decrease in albumin, other cations bound to albumin will also increase or decrease (e.g., magnesium and zinc).

Serum levels of phosphorus, alkaline phosphatase, urea nitrogen, creatinine, electrolytes, and magnesium outside the reference ranges favor a pathologic cause for an elevated calcium level. Consider that hypercalcemia may be caused by hyperlipoproteinemia or hyperproteinemia.

3. If hypercalcemia is documented by at least three serum calcium measurements and drugs are not the cause, consider the differential diagnosis as follows:

Severe hypercalcemia (>14 mg/dl [3.49 mmol/L]) favors nonparathyroid causes, usually cancer. Milder serum calcium elevations are typically seen in hyperparathyroidism. A diagnostic rule of thumb is that hypercalcemia that lasts more than a year without signs of primary cancer (or another identifiable cause) is caused by parathyroid disease.

The ratio of serum chloride to phosphorus is helpful. In hyperparathyroid patients, chloride values are high (mean of 107 mEq/L [107 mmol/L]), and the chloride-phosphorus ratios range from 32 to 80, with 96% of values higher than 33. In patients with hypercalcemia from other causes, the chloride values are lower (mean of 98 mEq/L [98 mmol/L]), the phosphorus measurement is higher (mean of 4.5 mg/dl [1.45 mmol/L]), and the chloride-phosphorus ratios range from 18 to 32, with 92% of values lower than 30.

If the hypercalcemia is accompanied by an elevated alkaline phosphatase, the differential diagnosis includes hyperparathyroidism, hyperthyroidism, osteoblastic bone lesions, and malignancy. Alkaline phosphatase is not elevated in multiple myeloma. A serum alkaline phosphatase greater than twice the upper reference limit is unlikely to indicate uncomplicated primary hyperparathyroidism. A decreased serum alkaline phosphatase may occur in hypervitaminosis D related to an increased phosphorus.

Elevation of serum urea nitrogen and creatinine may suggest the nephropathy of mild hyyperparathyroidism.

Serum potassium levels may be low in patients with hypercalcemia (32%). Since patients with cancer tend to have higher serum calcium levels and the serum potassium varies inversely with the serum calcium, there is a higher prevalence of hypokalemia (52%) in patients with cancer.

A low urinary calcium (usually <60 mg/24 hr) (1.50 mmol/24 hr) is the diagnostic hallmark of familial hypocalciuric hypercalcemia, an autosomal dominant syndrome. The serum magnesium level may be elevated. If a low urinary calcium is found, this diagnosis should be considered, and family members should be screened for hypercalcemia.

Additional studies to consider include serum calcitriol (vitamin D), immunoreactive parathyroid hormone (iPTH), and urinary cyclic adenosine monophosphate (cAMP). An elevated iPTH level is consistent with the diagnosis of hyperparathyroidism, but measurement of iPTH is complicated, and only laboratories with proven proficiency should be used. Up to now, different kinds of iPTH assays have been available, depending on which part of the PTH molecule the test antibody was directed against (i.e., n-terminal, c-terminal, or midmolecular region). New assays have been developed that recognize intact PTH, and these new assays will probably emerge as the gold standard. In the meantime, clinical assessment with routine laboratory tests plays a pivotal role in the assessment of patients with hypercalcemia.[5,6]

4.   If additional calcium measurements are normal and the elevated calcium can be explained on the basis of drug therapy, improper specimen collection and handling, or laboratory error, conclude that the patient does not have a pathologic cause for hypercalcemia.

5.   In patients with hypercalcemia, the following additional abnormal laboratory test results may occur:

HEMATOLOGY

• Anemia and an elevated erythrocyte sedimentation rate (ESR) suggest a nonparathyroid cause, particularly malignancy, although these findings may occur in primary hyperparathyroidism.

CHEMISTRY

• Elevated urea nitrogen, creatinine, and uric acid secondary to nephropathy. Uric acid may be elevated in malignancy because of high cell turnover and proliferation.
• Hyperchloremia secondary to decreased bicarbonate. Hyperchloremic metabolic acidosis favors primary hyperparathyroidism. Hypochloremic metabolic alkalosis favors metastatic cancer.

- Depressed total CO_2 because parathyroid hormone increases urinary bicarbonate excretion.
- Hyperphosphatemia without renal failure suggests a nonparathyroid cause. Hypophosphatemia (when dietary phosphorus is adequate and patient is not taking oral phosphate binding agents) favors primary hyperparathyroidism but can occur in malignancy.
- Elevated serum transaminase (AST or SGOT) and alkaline phosphatase (ALP) tests with granulomatous hepatitis, for example, sarcoidosis.
- Elevated lactate dehydrogenase (LD) caused by high malignant cell turnover and proliferation.
- Elevated alkaline phosphatase (ALP) occurs more often in malignancy and is unlikely in primary hyperparathyroidism in the absence of osteitis fibrosa cystica. The Regan and Nagao isoenzyme may occur in patients with bronchogenic carcinoma.
- Polyclonal hypergammaglobulinemia favors sarcoidosis but has been seen in primary hyperparathyroidism.

REFERENCES

1. Fallon MA, Arvan DA: Hypercalcemia. In Griner PF, Panzer RJ, Greenland P: Clinical Diagnosis and the Laboratory: Logical Strategies for Common Medical Problems. Chicago, Year Book Medical Publishers, Inc, 1986, p 531.
2. Goldsmith RS: Hypercalcemia (hyperparathyroidism). In Cutler P: Problem Solving in Clinical Medicine: From Data to Diagnosis, 2nd ed. Baltimore, Williams & Wilkins, 1985, p 454.
3. Gray TA, Paterson CR: The clinical value of ionized calcium assays. Ann Clin Biochem 25:210, 1988.
4. Heath H, Hodgson SF, Kennedy MA: Primary hyperparathyroidism: Incidence, morbidity, and potential economic impact in a community. N Engl J Med 302:189, 1980.
5. Lufkin EG, Kao PC, Heath H: Parathyroid hormone radioimmunoassays in the differential diagnosis of hypercalcemia due to primary hyperparathyroidism or malignancy. Ann Intern Med 106:559, 1987.
6. Measuring the PTH level. Lancet 1:94, 1988.
7. Sherwood LM: Diagnosis and management of primary hyperparathyroidism. Hosp Pract 23:9, 1988.
8. Toffaletti JG: Ionized calcium. Lab Report for Physicians 11:5, 1989.
9. Walmsley RN, White GH: Hypercalcemia. In Pocket Diagnostic Clinical Chemistry. Melbourne, Blackwell Scientific Publications, 1985, p 63.

HYPOCALCEMIA AND HYPOPARATHYROIDISM

Hypocalcemia may be caused by a relative or absolute deficiency of parathyroid hormone (PTH). Adequate vitamin D is also important. An absolute deficiency of PTH can occur because of loss of parathyroid tissue after parathyroidectomy or thyroidectomy or idiopathically. A relative deficiency can occur from resistance to PTH either congenitally or secondary to hypomagnesemia, chronic renal failure, malabsorption, or anticonvulsant therapy. Miscellaneous causes of hypocalcemia, where the mechanism is not completely clear, include acute pancreatitis, osteoblastic metastases, and rhabdomyolysis. Clinical findings of hypocalcemia may occur acutely (perioral paresthesias, restlessness, depression, Chvostek's or Trousseau's sign) or chronically (fatigue, cramps, muscle aches).[2-4]

1. In patients with clinical findings of hypocalcemia or if an individual is found to have a low serum calcium level, request at least three measurements of serum calcium together with a complete blood count (CBC), serum albumin and globulins by electrophoresis, phosphorus, magnesium, alkaline phosphatase, urea nitrogen, creatinine, and electrolytes. In certain circumstances, measurement of serum ionized calcium may be helpful.

Measurements of calcium, albumin, and phosphorus are useful to verify the hypocalcemia and to attempt to further classify it. Serum urea nitrogen, creatinine, and electrolytes can help to assess renal function, and a CBC and an alkaline phosphatase may provide valuable clues concerning the presence of malignancy.

The specimen collection issues are the same as for hypercalcemia.

2. Evaluate the tests.

The test considerations are the same as for hypercalcemia.

3. If hypocalcemia is documented by at least three serum calcium measurements and drugs are not the cause, consider the differential diagnosis as follows:

A common cause of a low serum calcium from hypoparathyroidism is prior thyroid surgery. Hypoparathyroidism may also occur idiopathically. In addition to a deficiency of (PTH), a low serum calcium may be caused by failure of the kidneys to respond to normal amounts of PTH, so-called pseudohypoparathyroidism. In either hypoparathyroidism or pseudohypoparathyroidism, the phosphorus is high. Both hypomagnesemia and hypermagnesemia can impair PTH secretion, causing hypocalcemia. Renal failure is perhaps the most common of all causes of hypocalcemia: the serum urea nitrogen, creatinine, and phosphorus are all elevated. In intestinal malabsorption, defective absorption of both calcium and vitamin D can occur, resulting in hypocalcemia. Miscellaneous causes of hypocalcemia include acute pancreatitis, osteoblastic metastatic bone disease, excessive transfusion with citrated blood, and rhabdomyolysis-induced renal failure. After parathyroid surgery, hypocalcemia may be caused by the hungry bone syndrome in which remineralization of the skeleton causes hypocalcemia and hypophosphatemia, often with tetany, requiring vigorous, prolonged calcium and vitamin D therapy.[1]

4. If the low serum calcium can be explained on the basis of drug therapy, improper specimen collection and handling, or laboratory error, conclude that the patient does not have a pathologic cause for hypocalcemia.

A low serum calcium may be caused by a testing problem, or it may be related to a low serum albumin. Certain drugs, such as phenytoin and other anticonvulsant medications, have been implicated as a cause of vitamin D deficiency and borderline-low serum calcium levels. It is important to identify these causes of a low serum calcium, so that a needless search for some underlying disease or disorder can be averted.

5.   In patients with hypoparathyroidism, the following additional abnormal laboratory test results may occur:

• Increased creatine kinase (CK), aspartate aminotransferase (AST or SGOT), and lactate dehydrogenase (LD) caused by myopathy

REFERENCES

1.   Brasier AR, Nussbaum SR: Hungry bone syndrome: Clinical and biochemical predictors of its occurrence after parathyroid surgery. Am J Med 84:654, 1988.
2.   Nusynowitz ML, Frame B, Kolb FO: The spectrum of the hypoparathyroid states: A classification based on physiologic principles. Medicine 55:105, 1976.
3.   Schneider AB, Sherwood LM: Pathogenesis and management of hypoparathyroidism and other hypocalcemic disorders. Metabolism 24:871, 1975.
4.   Walmsley RN, White GH: Hypocalcemia. In Pocket Diagnostic Clinical Chemistry. Melbourne, Blackwell Scientific Publications, 1985, p 65.

DIABETES MELLITUS

Surveys in the United States reveal that 2% to 4% of the population has documented diabetes and that a similar percentage has compromised glucose tolerance that is undetected. With advancing age, an even greater proportion of the population develops diabetes. The strategy that follows is recommended by the National Diabetes Data Group.[3] There are three different tactics for diagnosing diabetes. One is to find a significantly elevated serum glucose in the presence of obvious features of the disease; the second is to discover an elevated fasting serum glucose with or without clinical findings; and the third is to find an abnormal oral glucose tolerance test. Use of this strategy will eliminate many unnecessary glucose tolerance tests. Although screening for gestational diabetes is beneficial, routine screening for diabetes in the nonpregnant adult is not very productive.[2-4,6,7]

1.   In patients with obvious features of diabetes, such as rapid weight loss, polyuria, polydipsia, and ketonuria, immediately measure serum glucose — fasting or nonfasting. A value above 200 mg/dl (11.10 mmol/L) is diagnostic of diabetes.

The importance of obtaining a good blood sample for analysis cannot be overemphasized. At room temperature glucose is metabolized in a tube of blood at approximately 7 mg/dl/hr (0.39 mmol/L/hr). At 4°C the rate is approximately 2 mg/dl/hr (0.11 mmol/L/hr). Glucose is metabolized even more rapidly in blood taken from patients with leukocytosis/leukemia. This metabolic loss of glucose can be prevented by promptly (within ½ hour) separating the serum from the blood cells or by using collection tubes containing fluoride.

2. In patients with findings of subclinical diabetes such as unusual infections, worsening vision, or periodontal disease, measure a fasting serum glucose (morning sample after a 10-hour fast). A value greater than 140 mg/dl (7.77 mmol/L) is diagnostic. Do not test patients who are acutely ill. Routine screening for diabetes in the nonpregnant adult is not very productive.[6]

A fasting serum glucose above 140 mg/dl (7.77 mmol/L) supports the diagnosis of diabetes and makes an oral glucose tolerance test unnecessary. A second fasting glucose above 140 mg/dl (7.77 mmol/L) is required to actually make the diagnosis. However, a fasting serum glucose below 140 mg/dl (7.77 mmol/L) but above 115 mg/dl (6.38 mmol/L) does not exclude diabetes, because it is not as sensitive a test for diabetes as is an oral glucose tolerance test. A fasting serum glucose below 115 mg/dl excludes diabetes. Acute illness can affect serum glucose levels and cause misleading results.

3. If the fasting serum glucose is 115 to 140 mg/dl (6.38 to 7.77 mmol/L), perform a morning oral glucose tolerance test. Do not test patients who are acutely ill.

A glucose tolerance test has greater sensitivity than a fasting serum glucose level, but unless the patient is properly prepared, overdiagnosis can be a problem. Overdiagnosis can adversely affect insurance rates, employability, and mental health. The test should not be done during an acute medical or surgical illness in the hospital. It should only be performed on healthy, ambulatory patients who are not taking drugs that affect glucose tolerance.[4]

Since patients with type I diabetes, or insulin-dependent diabetes mellitus (IDDM), typically have hyperglycemia, ketosis, and acidosis, most patients tested will have type II, or non-insulin-dependent diabetes mellitus (NIDDM; 85% to 90% of diabetics) or impaired glucose tolerance (IGT). Pregnant patients require a special glucose tolerance test.

Alternative methods to determine glucose tolerance, such as measurement of a postprandial or random serum glucose or performance of a glucose tolerance test regardless of the time of the last meal, are not recommended as definitive procedures.

The oral glucose tolerance test may be compromised if the protocol is not closely followed and the results correctly interpreted.[8] Perform the oral glucose tolerance test in the morning after the person has fasted at least 10 hours but not more than 16 hours. The subject should not be ill or taking a medication known to affect the blood sugar and should have had normal physical activity and carbohydrate intake greater than 150 g/day for a least 3 days before the glucose tolerance test. The individual should remain seated and should not eat, smoke, or drink coffee, tea, or alcohol during the test. First, draw a fasting blood glucose sample, and afterward give 75 g of glucose orally (challenge dose for children is 1.75 g/kg of ideal body weight up to 75 g). The oral glucose solution should be ingested in less than 5 minutes, and the clock starts running when the patient begins to drink. Then draw blood samples every 30 minutes for 2 hours.

The following drugs and chemical agents are known to affect glucose tolerance (see reference 3 for additional drugs)[3,4]:

Diuretics and antihypertensive agents
- Chlorthalidone
- Clonidine
- Diazoxide
- Furosemide
- Thiazides

Hormonally active agents
- Corticotropin
- Glucagon
- Glucocorticoids
- Oral contraceptives
- Somatotropin
- Thyroid hormones

Psychoactive agents
- Chlorprothixene
- Haloperidol
- Lithium carbonate
- Phenothiazines
- Tricyclic antidepressants

Catecholamines and other neurologically active agents
- Epinephrine
- Isoproterenol
- Levodopa
- Norepinephrine
- Phenytoin

Analgesic, antipyretic, and antiinflammatory agents

Antineoplastic agents
- Alloxan
- L-Asparaginase
- Streptozocin

Miscellaneous agents
- Encainide[5]
- Isoniazid
- Nicotinic acid

4. Evaluate the tests.

It is essential to use a laboratory with an accurately standardized glucose method. Enzymatic methods for measuring serum glucose such as hexokinase or glucose oxidase are best, because they give the most accurate results. Reduction methods such as ferricyanide and neocuproine are obsolete and tend to overestimate the serum glucose value because of non-glucose-reducing substances in the blood. In uremia, serious errors can occur using reduction methods because of overestimation of serum glucose up to 40 mg/dl (2.22 mmol/L) as a result of uric acid and creatinine. Patients taking vitamin C have depressed serum glucose levels when measured with the glucose oxidase method.

Consider measuring the fasting serum glucose before doing the glucose tolerance test. If the fasting serum glucose level is greater than 140 mg/dl (7.77 mmol/L), the diagnosis of diabetes is supported and a glucose tolerance test is unnecessary. If the fasting serum glucose level is less than 115 mg/dl (6.38 mmol/L), the diagnosis of diabetes is excluded. If the fasting serum glucose level is 115 to 140 mg/dl (6.38 to 7.77 mmol/L), proceed with the oral glucose tolerance test.

POSITIVE ORAL GLUCOSE TOLERANCE TEST

TIME	VALUE
Fasting	<140 mg/dl (7.77 mmol/L)
½ hr	Both 2-hr sample and at least
1 hr	one other sample must
1½ hr	be >200 mg/dl
2 hr	(11.10 mmol/L)

IMPAIRED ORAL GLUCOSE TOLERANCE TEST

TIME	VALUE
Fasting	<140 mg/dl (7.77 mmol/L)
½ hr	2-hr sample must be
1 hr	140–200 mg/dl
	(7.77–11.10 mmol/L)
1½ hr	and at least one other
2 hr	sample must be >200 mg/dl
	(11.10 mmol/L)

5. If the diagnosis of diabetes is supported by an elevated fasting serum glucose level or a positive tolerance test, confirm the diagnosis by obtaining one or more additional positive results, such as another elevated fasting serum glucose level or another positive oral glucose tolerance test result.

In light of the many factors other than diabetes that elevate fasting serum glucose and impair glucose tolerance, it is imperative that an elevated fasting serum glucose or a positive oral glucose tolerance test be demonstrated on more than one occasion before a clinical diagnosis of diabetes is made.

6. If the diagnosis of impaired glucose tolerance is supported by the oral glucose tolerance test, reexamine the patient yearly.

Individuals with impaired glucose tolerance may develop overt diabetes (at the rate of 1% to 5% per year), revert to normal glucose tolerance, or remain in the intermediate range. Persons with impaired glucose tolerance rarely have clinically significant microvascular disease.

7. If the diagnosis of diabetes is confirmed, begin therapy and monitor the patient's glucose homeostasis using measurements of serum glucose, urinary glucose, and hemoglobin A_{1c}.

If the diagnosis of diabetes mellitus is confirmed, begin therapy and monitor the patient's glucose homeostasis using measurements of serum glucose, urinary glucose, and hemoglobin A_{1c} as appropriate. Self-glucose monitoring is a method for diabetics to achieve and maintain normal serum glucose (tight control) that is becoming more popular. It is particularly useful in patients who are prone to severe hypoglycemic reactions, such as certain women during pregnancy. Assessment of glycosuria is not very helpful in attempting to maintain the serum glucose near normal. This is because the renal threshold for serum glucose in normal persons is approximately 180 to 200 mg/dl (9.99 to 11.10 mmol/L) and this threshold may increase with renal disease. In the appropriate circumstances, the measurement of ketones in the urine remains important.[7]

The goals for serum glucose control in healthy diabetic patients below 65 years old follow (in older patients, goals may be shifted upward)[II]:

Fasting and preprandial
    Ideal: 70–100 mg/dl (3.89–5.55 mmol/L)
    Acceptable: 60–130 mg/dl (3.33–7.22 mmol/L)
Postprandial
    Ideal: <160 mg/dl (8.88 mmol/L)
    Acceptable: <200 mg/dl (11.10 mmol/L)
3:00 AM
    Ideal: >65 mg/dl (3.61 mmol/L)
    Acceptable: >65 mg/dl (3.61 mmol/L)

Hemoglobin A_{1c} is a test that complements serum glucose monitoring. When serum glucose is high, it irreversibly combines with hemoglobin to form hemoglobin A_{1c}, and hemoglobin A_{1c} reflects the patient's average serum glucose for about 2 to 3 months before testing. It can also be useful to differentiate stress hyperglycemia, such as occurs with a myocardial infarction, from chronic hyperglycemia. In stress hyperglycemia, hemoglobin A_{1c} is normal, whereas in chronic hyperglycemia it is elevated. There is a strong relationship between hyperglycemia, elevated hemoglobin A_{1c}, and the incidence and progression of diabetic retinopathy.[1]

In healthy, nondiabetic individuals, about 5% to 7% of blood hemoglobin is in the form of hemoglobin A_{1c}. Mild hyperglycemia is associated with a hemoglobin A_{1c} concentration of 8% to 10% and severe hyperglycemia with a hemoglobin A_{1c} concentration as high as 20%. Hemoglobin A_{1c} may also be elevated secondary to iron deficiency. Be careful to use your laboratory's normal range for hemoglobin A_{1c}, because the normal range may vary with different measurement techniques.[V]

8. In diabetic patients, the following additional abnormal laboratory test results may occur:

HEMATOLOGY

- Elevated platelet count

CHEMISTRY

- Elevated urea nitrogen, creatinine, and uric acid with renal failure. Elevated glucose and acetone can interfere with creatinine methodology.
- Hypouricemia caused by hyperuricosuria.
- Hyponatremia caused by hyperglycemia.
- Hypocalcemia, hypokalemia, hyponatremia, and hypochloremia from osmotic diuresis caused by hyperglycemia.
- Hyperkalemia related to metabolic acidosis.
- Depressed total CO_2 from ketoacidosis.
- Hypercalcemia from hyperalbuminemia with dehydration.
- Hyperphosphatemia caused by glucose intolerance with hyperglycemia.

- Elevated creatine kinase (CK), lactate dehydrogenase (LH), and transaminase levels (AST or SGOT and ALT or SGPT) caused by effects on skeletal muscle and fatty liver.
- Elevated alkaline phosphatase.
- Hyperproteinemia and hyperalbuminemia caused by dehydration.
- Hypoalbuminemia.
- Hypercholesterolemia and hypertriglyceridemia caused by disturbed carbohydrate metabolism.

REFERENCES

1. Klein R, Klein BEK, Moss SE, et al: Glycosylated hemoglobin predicts the incidence and progression of diabetic retinopathy. JAMA 260:2864, 1988.
2. Moreno CA: Glycosuria (diabetes mellitus). In Cutler P: Problem Solving in Clinical Medicine: From Data to Diagnosis. Baltimore, Williams & Wilkins, 1985, p 273.
3. National Diabetes Data Group: Classification and diagnosis of diabetes mellitus and other categories of glucose intolerance. Diabetes 28:1039, 1979.
4. Nelson RL: Oral and glucose tolerance test: Indications and limitations. Mayo Clin Proc 63:263, 1988.
5. Salerno DM, Fifield J, Krejci J, et al: Encainide-induced hyperglycemia. Am J Med 84:39, 1988.
6. Singer DE, Samet JH, Coley CM, et al: Screening for diabetes mellitus. Ann Intern Med 109:639, 1988.
7. Watts NB: Disorders of Glucose Metabolism. Chicago, American Society of Clinical Pathologists Press, 1987.
8. Wiener K: The oral glucose tolerance test—an assessment of the quality of its performance. Ann Clin Biochem 24:440, 1987.

DIABETES MELLITUS IN PREGNANCY

Gestational diabetes is defined as carbohydrate intolerance of variable severity with onset or first recognition during the current pregnancy. It occurs in 2.4% of all pregnancies in the United States and accounts for 86,000 cases annually. Maternal diabetes is associated with a variety of fetal and neonatal abnormalities including a heavy-for-date baby, hypoglycemia, respiratory distress, and congenital anomalies. The strategy that follows is recommended by the National Diabetes Data Group[2] and the Second International Workshop-Conference on Gestational Diabetes.[5] The special pregnancy oral glucose tolerance test is different from the one used in nonpregnant individuals. Moreover, the strategy recognizes that the woman with gestational diabetes must be reclassified after the pregnancy is over. Screening for gestational diabetes is clearly beneficial.[1-5]

1. Screen all pregnant women for gestational diabetes mellitus (GDM) between the twenty-fourth and twenty-eighth weeks of pregnancy with a 50 g oral glucose load without regard to the time of the last meal or the time of day, and measure serum glucose at 1 hour. If a pregnant woman

has a history of diabetes, screen her in the same manner at the time of the initial visit. Do not use hemoglobin A₁c for screening.

Twenty-four to twenty-eight weeks is the optimal time for screening, since at this time the frequency of GDM peaks and there is still sufficient time for appropriate therapy.[3]

The specimen collection and handling and methodologic considerations are the same as for diagnosing diabetes in nonpregnant individuals.

2.   If the 1-hour serum glucose level is above 140 mg/dl (7.77 mmol/L), perform the 100 g pregnancy oral glucose tolerance test.

Clinical features that suggest GDM include glycosuria, a family history of diabetes, a history of stillbirth or spontaneous abortion, a previous fetal malformation, a previous heavy-for-date baby, obesity, high maternal age, or parity of five or more.

Gestational diabetes is restricted to pregnant women in whom the onset or recognition of diabetes or impaired glucose tolerance occurs during pregnancy. Diabetic women who become pregnant are not included in this category.

Clinical recognition of GDM is important because (1) in a setting where high-risk pregnancies can be managed effectively, therapy can prevent much of the associated perinatal morbidity and mortality, and (2) these women are at higher risk of developing diabetes 5 to 10 years after parturition.

Perform the oral glucose tolerance test the same way as in screening for diabetes in the nonpregnant individual with these exceptions. Give 100 g glucose orally instead of 75 g and draw blood samples every hour for 3 hours instead of every 30 minutes for 2 hours.

The specimen collection issues are the same as for diabetes mellitus in the preceding problem.

3.   Evaluate the tests.

The methodologic considerations are the same as for diabetes mellitus.

**POSITIVE ORAL GLUCOSE TOLERANCE
TEST IN PREGNANCY**

TIME	VALUE*
Fasting	>105 mg/dl (5.83 mmol/L)
1 hr	>190 mg/dl (10.55 mmol/L)
2 hr	>165 mg/dl (9.16 mmol/L)
3 hr	>145 mg/dl (8.05 mmol/L)

*Any two or more values exceeding these concentrations are diagnostic.

4.   If the oral glucose tolerance is positive, it supports the diagnosis of GDM, but reexamine the patient after the pregnancy is over using the strategy for the nonpregnant adult.

After pregnancy terminates, the woman must be reexamined to determine whether she is normal, diabetic, or impaired in her glucose homeostasis. A woman with GDM who reverts to normal is classified as a previous abnormality of glucose tolerance. In the majority of patients with GDM, glucose tolerance returns to normal postpartum, and the subject can be reclassified as having a previous abnormality of glucose tolerance. About 40% of women with GDM will become diabetic within 15 years after delivery, and the risk increases with obesity. Once a woman has had GDM, a 90% chance exists for recurrence with future pregnancies.[3]

REFERENCES

1. Glucose tolerance in pregnancy—the who and how of testing. Lancet 2:1173, 1988.
2. National Diabetes Data Group: Classification and diagnosis of diabetes mellitus and other categories of glucose intolerance. Diabetes 28:1039, 1979.
3. Nelson RL: Oral glucose tolerance tests: Indications and limitations. Mayo Clin Proc 63:263, 1988.
4. Singer DE, Samet JH, Coley CM, et al: Screening for diabetes mellitus. Ann Intern Med 109:639, 1988.
5. Summary and recommendations of the Second International Workshop-Conference on Gestational Diabetes Mellitus. Diabetes 34(suppl 2):123, 1985.

TRUE HYPOGLYCEMIA AND THE IDIOPATHIC POSTPRANDIAL SYNDROME

Physicians are always alert to clinical findings that suggest hypoglycemia, because they know that hypoglycemia poses a threat to the integrity of the central nervous system. The brain depends on glucose as its primary energy substrate and cannot use free fatty acids as other tissues do. Low serum glucose not only impairs neural function, but if the serum glucose level is profoundly and persistently depressed, irreversible brain damage and even death may ensue. The strategy for the differential diagnosis of hypoglycemia depends on documenting a low serum glucose in the presence of clinical findings and noting whether the patient is in the fasting or postprandial state. In contrast to true hypoglycemia, in which the serum glucose is truly low, the idiopathic postprandial syndrome (formerly called reactive hypoglycemia or functional hypoglycemia) is a situation in which a postprandial patient has clinical findings that suggest hypoglycemia and the serum glucose is normal.[3,5–8,11]

1. In patients with clinical findings of hypoglycemia, measure serum glucose. Glucose should be administered following blood withdrawal to any patient suspected of being hypoglycemic.

The study of any patient with signs and symptoms suggesting hypoglycemia begins by measuring serum glucose. If the signs and symptoms are serious (e.g., confusion or coma), an intravenous administration of a bolus of 25 or 50 g glucose as a 50% solution followed by constant infusion of glucose until the patient is able to eat a meal is appropriate. Findings such as sweating, tremor, tachycardia, anxiety, and hunger without central nervous system symptoms and signs can be treated with oral carbohydrates and do not require parenteral glucose.

The true hypoglycemia syndrome refers to the presence of adrenergic or neuroglycopenic signs and symptoms in the presence of a low serum glucose concentration—generally below 40 mg/dl (2.22 mmol/L)—where the signs and symptoms can be relieved by the administration of glucose. This constellation of findings is sometimes referred to as Whipple's triad. The adrenergic signs and symptoms are those induced by epinephrine secretion and consist of sweating, tremor, tachycardia, anxiety, and hunger. Neuroglycopenic findings are caused by low central nervous system glucose and consist of dizziness, headache, clouded vision, blunted mental acuity, confusion, abnormal behavior, convusions, and coma. Persistent, very low central nervous system glucose levels can cause features of decortication or decerebration as well as focal abnormalities, particularly hemiplegia. Without glucose administration, these defects may become permanent. Interestingly, the peripheral nervous system is seldom affected by hypoglycemia.

The idiopathic postprandial syndrome is a term applied to the adrenergic signs and symptoms (often reduced by glucose administration) that occur in many individuals 2 to 5 hours after a meal. Generally, if serum glucose is measured, these individuals do not have hypoglycemia. Since the cause of the adrenergic findings is frequently unclear, the term "idiopathic postprandial syndrome" has been suggested. For every 50 to 100 patients with "normoglycemic" reactive hypoglycemia, there may be one with true hypoglycemia.

The 5-hour oral glucose tolerance test has been widely used to document hypoglycemia in patients with postprandial adrenergic signs and symptoms. Since healthy persons may have hypoglycemia without symptoms and symptomatic persons usually have normoglycemia, the oral glucose tolerance test, including the 5-hour oral glucose tolerance test, should be abandoned as a tool for diagnosis. *The only unequivocal diagnostic test for true hypoglycemia is a low serum glucose concentration during spontaneously developed symptoms.*[II]

In the workup of a patient with hypoglycemia, a detailed history is essential and should include every medication (prescription and nonprescription), as well as alcohol ingestion. For patients who have underlying disease, the results of the history and physical examination should determine the direction of the investigation.

One must be constantly alert to artifactual hypoglycemia. Serum should be promptly separated from blood cells or blood should be preserved with fluoride, since blood cells will metabolize glucose and lower the serum glucose concentration. This effect is greatly accelerated in polycythemia, leukemia, and leukocytosis.

2. Evaluate the serum glucose result.

A low serum glucose level is generally considered to be one that is below 40 mg/dl (2.22 mmol/L). Normally, at glucose levels of 40 mg/dl or less, little or no insulin is released. Remember that the glucose level may be falsely depressed in improperly handled specimens and that vitamin C ingestion may depress values measured with the glucose oxidase method. The methodologic considerations are the same as for diagnosing diabetes.

Serum glucose levels do not always correlate with an individual's signs and symptoms. Symptoms of hypoglycemia usually occur at serum glucose levels below 40 mg/dl (2.22 mmol/L), but some persons show no findings with levels as low as 30 mg/dl (1.67 mmol/L). Other persons may show findings at levels up to 100 mg/dl (5.55 mmol/L) when the serum glucose rapidly falls from a previously high level. Adrenergic signs and symptoms seem to be related to a rapidly falling glucose level. If glucose falls rapidly but central nervous system levels remain adequate, adrenergic findings may occur in the absence of neuroglycopenic findings. If the glucose level falls slowly to very low levels, neuroglycopenic findings may occur in the absence of adrenergic findings.[V]

3.   If a patient has a normal serum glucose level in the postprandial state, consider the idiopathic postprandial syndrome. Never use the oral glucose tolerance test to evaluate the idiopathic postprandial syndrome (reactive hypoglycemia).

In healthy individuals, ingestion of a meal provokes a rise in serum glucose and a brisk insulin release followed by a falling serum glucose and a decrease in insulin. Frequently, the falling glucose level drops below baseline, even below 40 mg/dl (2.22 mmol/L), but these persons usually have no symptoms. Insulin is the primary hypoglycemic hormone. Other hormones that affect serum glucose tend to elevate the serum level (i.e., cortisol, growth hormone, glucagon, catecholamines).

Patients in the postprandial state with clinical findings suggestive of hypoglycemia may or may not have a low serum glucose. If the patient has adrenergic signs and symptoms and the serum glucose is normal, then the diagnosis is the idiopathic postprandial syndrome. Treatment is controversial; however, a high-protein, low-carbohydrate diet is frequently prescribed for patients with the idiopathic postprandial syndrome and may relieve symptoms.

4.   If a patient has a low serum glucose in the postprandial state, consider the following causes of postprandial hypoglycemia:

- Alimentary hypoglycemia
- Hereditary fructose intolerance
- Galactosemia
- Leucine sensitivity
- Idiopathic hypoglycemia

ALIMENTARY HYPOGLYCEMIA

Alimentary hypoglycemia is the most common cause of postprandial hypoglycemia. After certain procedures, such as gastrectomy, gastrojejunostomy, pyloroplasty, or vagotomy, patients may have rapid postprandial gastric emptying with rapid absorption of glucose and excessive release of insulin. Since blood glucose levels tend to fall faster than insulin levels, hypoglycemia may ensue.

OTHER CAUSES OF POSTPRANDIAL HYPOGLYCEMIA

In certain children with fructose intolerance or galactosemia, ingestion of fructose or galactose causes hypoglycemia. Rarely, leucine can cause hypoglycemia in susceptible infants. True postprandial hypoglycemia of unknown cause or idiopathic hypoglycemia in which the patient has adrenergic signs and symptoms relieved by glucose administration is rare.

5.   If a patient has a low serum glucose in the fasting state, consider the following causes of fasting hypoglycemia[3]:

Hyperinsulinism
> Too much insulin in a diabetic patient
> Islet cell hyperplasia/tumor
> Factitious administration of insulin/sulfonylureas

Drugs
> Alcohol
> Salicylates in children
> Propranolol
> Disopyramide (Norpace)
> Sulfamethoxazole-trimethoprim (Bactrim, Septra) in renal failure
> Pentamidine (Pentam) and quinine when used to treat cerebral malaria
> Chlorpropamide (may stimulate beta cells, producing hyperinsulinemia)[4]
> Miscellaneous drugs

Acquired liver disease
> Hepatic congestion
> Severe hepatitis
> Cirrhosis
> Secondary to uremia

Hormone deficiencies
> Hypopituitarism
> Adrenal insufficiency

Extrapancreatic tumors
> Sarcomas
> Carcinomas of liver, gastrointestinal tract, and adrenal gland

Substrate deficiency
> Severe malnutrition
> Late pregnancy

Enzyme defects
> Glucose-6-phosphatase
> Pyruvate carboxylase

Insulin antibodies

Miscellaneous disorders
> Diffuse carcinomatosis
> Rampant leukemia

There are many causes of hypoglycemia in the fasting state that lower the blood glucose level either by increasing the utilization of glucose in the peripheral tissues or decreasing the availability of glucose. For example, hyperinsulinism, whether from exogenous insulin or an insulinoma, causes hypoglycemia by increasing the tissue utilization of glucose. On the other hand, alcohol causes hypoglycemia in fasting patients by inhibiting gluconeogenesis.

HYPERINSULINISM

Too much insulin in a diabetic who is taking insulin is perhaps the most common cause of fasting hypoglycemia.[1] The diagnosis is obvious.

Hypoglycemia secondary to islet cell hyperplasis or tumor may be provoked by fasting. Start with a 6- to 8-hour overnight fast but remember that a 48- to 64-hour fast may be required (exercise such as walking up and down stairs for an hour can help provoke hypoglycemia). Thirty-five percent will become hypoglycemic in 12 hours, 75% in 24 hours, and over 90% in 48 hours. Episodes of confusion may occur either in the morning before breakfast or long after a meal and be aggravated by exercise. These episodes are relieved within minutes by glucose. A serum glucose level below 40 mg/dl (2.22 mmol/L) and clinical findings of hypoglycemia promptly relieved by glucose administration but not by a placebo are virtually diagnostic of islet cell tumor.

Patients with hypoglycemia secondary to islet cell lesions have inappropriately high serum insulin and C-peptide levels at the time of hypoglycemia, so insulin and C-peptide levels should be measured along with glucose levels (in vivo, proinsulin in the beta cell is cleaved to form insulin and C-peptide). Measurements of glucose and insulin should be done on several occasions. The diagnosis of insulinoma is supported when an inappropriately elevated serum insulin (>6 μU/ml) (>6 mIU/L) is present when the serum glucose level is below 60 mg/dl (3.33 mmol/L). An overnight fasting serum glucose level below 60 mg/dl in an adult is suspect, especially when accompanied by a higher than expected insulin level.

Overnight fasting serum glucose and insulin levels should be measured several times and ratios of insulin to glucose calculated. If these values are normal, other protocols involving longer fasts or fasts plus exerise are available. Provocative tests using tolbutamide, leucine, or glucagon are also available. If the test values indicate an islet cell tumor, angiography is useful to locate the tumor and radiographic scanning to look for possible metastases.

Factitious hypoglycemia caused by insulin administration can be diagnosed by measuring serum insulin and C-peptide. In factitious hypoglycemia the serum insulin level is elevated and the C-peptide level is low, because insulin is administered directly, instead of being produced in the islet beta cells where proinsulin normally gives rise to elevated serum levels of both insulin and C-peptide. When available, antiinsulin antibodies are the most helpful diagnostic test.[2] Nondiabetic persons who secretly take insulin or sulfonylureas are predominately women in the third and fourth decades of life who are employed in health-related occupations.

DRUGS

After liver glycogen is depleted by fasting, alcohol can induce hypoglycemia by inhibiting gluconeogenesis. It does this by blocking the normal pathway of gluconeogenesis from pyruvate. Even low levels of serum alcohol, as low as 25 mg/dl (5.4 mmol/L), cause hypoglycemia. Apparently, propranolol can also impair gluconeogenesis. Moreover, the adrenergic signs and symptoms of hypoglycemia may not occur with propranolol, because it is a beta blocker that blunts the effects of epinephrine. *In a patient receiving insulin and propranolol, the prolongation of the duration of hypoglycemia and the masking of the symptoms of hypoglycemia may be dangerous.*

The hypoglycemic effect of salicylates was recognized long ago. It is especially prevalent in children and may occur even at relatively low doses of the drug. This hypoglycemic effect of salicylates has been recently emphasized in the context of Reye's syndrome.

Since a number of drugs have been implicated in the etiology of hypoglycemia, the reader should consult the literature for additional information.

OTHER CAUSES OF FASTING HYPOGLYCEMIA

Acquired liver disease may cause hypoglycemia be interfering with glycogen stores, and the hypoglycemia of uremia has been attributed to secondary effects on the liver. Since certain hormones, such as growth hormone and cortisol, have a hyperglycemic effect, deficiency states such as hypopituitarism and adrenal insufficiency can result in hypoglycemia. The liver requires appropriate substrates and enzymes to ensure an adequate supply of blood glucose, and if these are missing, such as the substrate deficiency of malnutrition or a critical enzyme deficiency, hypoglycemia occurs. Large extrapancreatic tumors apparently cause hypoglycemia by overutilization of glucose. Perhaps this is also the mechanism in diffuse carcinomatosis and rampant leukemia. The mechanism by which insulin antibodies cause hypoglycemia is not well understood.

6.   In patients with hypoglycemia, the following additional abnormal laboratory test results may occur:

- Hypokalemia and hypophosphatemia caused by intracellular shift of potassium following administration of glucose and insulin

REFERENCES

1. Feingold KR: Hypoglycemia: A pitfall of insulin therapy (Medical Staff Conference). 139:688, 1983.
2. Grunsberger G, Weiner JL, Silverman R, et al: Factitious hypoglycemia due to surreptitious administration of insulin. Ann Intern Med 108:252, 1988.
3. Kitabchi AE, Goodman RC: Hypoglycemia, pathophysiology, and diagnosis. Hosp Pract 22:45, 1987.
4. Klonoff DC: Association of hyperinsulinemia with chlorpropamide toxicity. Am J Med 84:33, 1988.
5. Kudzma DJ: Weakness, anxiety, sweating (hypoglycemia). In Cutler P: Problem Solving in Clinical Medicine: From Data to Diagnosis, 2nd ed. Baltimore, Williams & Wilkins, 1985, p 278.
6. Nelson RL: Oral glucose tolerance test: Indications and limitations. Mayo Clin Proc 63:263, 1988.
7. Service FJ (ed): Hypoglycemic Disorders: Pathogenesis, Diagnosis, and Treatment. Boston, GK Hall, 1983.
8. Watts NB: Disorders of Glucose Metabolism. Chicago, American Society of Clinical Pathologists Press, 1987.

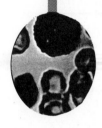

CHAPTER 9

CLASSIFYING ANEMIA BY
ERYTHROCYTE SIZE AND
RETICULOCYTE COUNT

THE COMMON ANEMIAS

INFECTIOUS MONONUCLEOSIS

HEMATOLOGIC DISORDERS

CLASSIFYING ANEMIA BY ERYTHROCYTE SIZE AND RETICULOCYTE COUNT

Anemia is defined as a diminished level of hemoglobin or hematocrit more than two standard deviations below the expected mean for age, sex, and physiologic state or as a gradual or sudden decline in hemoglobin or hematocrit from an established baseline level. Chronic anemia occurs in about 1% of men and about 10% of women. In the elderly, the prevalence may reach 10% to 15% in either sex. In the United States, in over 75% of cases, chronic anemia is caused by iron deficiency, chronic disease, or thalassemia. In a prospective study of patients admitted to the service of a university hospital, the rate of recognition of mild to moderate anemia by the patients' physicians was only 75%. Although the physician recognition rate for anemia increased with severity, it did not reach 100% until the hemoglobin was below 9 g/dl (90 g/L). Patients with chronic anemia may do surprisingly well until the hemoglobin falls to 6 to 8 g/dl (60 to 80 g/L) when symptoms appear with exercise or stress. When the hemoglobin falls below 6 g/dl (60 g/L), dyspnea, fatigue, and other symptoms occur. In acute anemia from blood loss or hemolysis, clinical findings are related to hypovolemia.[1-4]

1. In patients with clinical findings of anemia or if you wish to screen for anemia, request a complete blood count (CBC).

A CBC performed on an automated instrument is widely available and includes a hemoglobin, hematocrit, red cell indices, leukocytes—and sometimes platelets and an electronic differential as well. On the other hand, if a discrete hemoglobin or hematocrit measurement is available, you may wish to order only a hemoglobin or hematocrit.

2. If anemia is present, determine the reticulocyte count.

Normally, there are 1% to 1.5% reticulocytes in the peripheral blood, and a simple determination of the peripheral blood reticulocyte count is often sufficient; however, in some situations, such as the hemolytic anemias, it may be useful to determine the corrected absolute reticulocyte count. To calculate the total number of reticulocytes per cubic millimeter of blood (corrected absolute reticulocyte count) the percentage of reticulocytes must be corrected for maturation time and total red blood cell count as follows:[V]

$$\frac{\text{Percent reticulocytes on peripheral smear} \times \text{RBC count}}{\text{Reticulocyte maturation time}} = \text{Corrected absolute reticulocyte count}$$

The reference range for the corrected absolute reticulocyte count is

$$50,000/mm^3 \pm 25,000/mm^3$$

In percentages, a corrected reticulocyte count of less than 2% indicates reduced production of erythrocytes, and a corrected reticulocyte count greater than 2% indicates accelerated production of erythrocytes.[1]

3.   Then characterize the anemia as microcytic, macrocytic, or normocytic with or without reticulocytosis.

Classification of anemia according to erythrocyte size and reticulocytosis is a useful first step toward finding a cause. For example, iron deficiency anemia, thalassemia minor, and anemia of chronic disease often are seen as microcytic anemia without reticulocytosis, whereas anemia caused by folic acid or vitamin B_{12} deficiency is seen as macrocytic anemia without reticulocytosis. In contrast, hemolytic anemias typically show reticulocytosis.

REFERENCES

1. Hematology Subspecialty Committee: Medical Knowledge Self-Assessment Program VIII. Hematology. Philadelphia, American College of Physicians, 1988, p 461.
2. Self KG, Conrady MM, Eichner ER: Failure to diagnose anemia in medical patients: Is the traditional diagnosis of anemia a dying art? Am J Med 81:786, 1986.
3. Shapiro MF, Greenfield S: The complete blood count and leukocyte differential count. An approach to their rational application. In Sox HC (ed): Common Diagnostic Tests. Use and Interpretation. Philadelphia, American College of Physicians, 1987, p 133.
4. Wallerstein RO: Laboratory evaluation of anemia. West J Med 146:443, 1987.

THE COMMON ANEMIAS*

Like fever, anemia is a sign of disease, and although there are many different forms of anemia, iron deficiency anemia, thalassemia, and anemia of chronic disease account for more than 75% of cases of anemia in the United States. Other less frequent but important causes of anemia include sickle cell disease, aplasia, autoimmune hemolytic anemia, erythrocyte enzyme defects, and B_{12} and folate deficiency. This discussion will focus on iron deficiency anemia, beta-thalassemia minor, and anemia of chronic disease, which happen to be microcytic anemias, and will not cover other more unusual microcytic anemias, such as anemia of lead poisoning, congenital sideroblastic anemia, beta-thalassemia intermedia and major, and hemoglobin H or E disease.[1-11]

1.   In patients with microcytic anemia, assess the clinical findings; review or request a complete blood count (CBC), erythrocyte indices, and reticulocyte count; and examine the peripheral blood smear. Consider requesting a serum iron, total iron-binding capacity, ferritin, and, if

*Microcytic anemias without reticulocytosis.

appropriate, hemoglobin electrophoresis. If the red cell distribution width (RDW)* is available, it may be helpful in distinguishing iron deficiency anemia from anemia of chronic disease and beta-thalassemia.

Iron deficiency anemia, beta-thalassemia minor, and anemia of chronic disease are three common anemias characterized by erythrocytic microcytosis without reticulocytosis. This classification is not completely categorical. For example, anemia caused by iron deficiency and anemia of chronic disease may be normocytic; an additional confounding issue may be the presence of more than one cause for the anemia; for example, there is a high incidence of iron deficiency anemia in pernicious anemia.[2]

A practical approach in the absence of an obvious chronic disease is to initially determine whether the anemia is caused by iron deficiency. The serum iron and total iron-binding capacity are generally more easily available than the serum ferritin, and if these are diagnostic, there may be no need to measure serum ferritin. When the probability of uncomplicated anemia caused by iron deficiency is high on clinical grounds alone, the serum ferritin and percent saturation of transferrin are about equally useful in confirming the diagnosis of iron deficiency anemia, but when the clinical probability is low, ferritin is the better test.[5] Only two conditions other than iron deficiency anemia decrease ferritin levels: hypothyroidism and ascorbate deficiency.[3] Another approach to the diagnosis of iron deficiency anemia is a therapeutic trial: determine whether iron therapy produces a reticulocytosis. Clues to the diagnosis of beta-thalassemia minor are a normal RDW and a mean corpuscular volume (MCV) below 80 fl in patients with normal or borderline iron studies and no evidence of other causes of microcytosis.[4,7–11]

2. Evaluate the tests.

---

*The RDW measures variability of red cell size (anisocytosis) and is now calculated as part of a CBC on many automated counters.

REFERENCE RANGE VALUES[x]

TEST	SPECIMEN	REFERENCE RANGE (CONVENTIONAL)	REFERENCE RANGE (INTERNATIONAL)
Reticulocyte count	Whole blood (EDTA, heparin, or oxalate)	0.5–1.5% of erythrocytes	0.005–0.015 of erythrocytes
Iron	Serum	M*: 50–160 μg/dl F†: 40–150 μg/dl	8.95–28.64 μmol/L 7.16–26.85 μmol/L
Iron-binding capacity (TIBC)	Serum	250–400 μg/dl	44.75–71.60 μmol/L
Ferritin	Serum	M: 15–200 ng/ml F: 12–150 ng/ml	15–200 μg/L 12–150 μg/L

*Male.
†Female.

3. Interpret test results in the context of clinical findings.

THE COMMON ANEMIAS

	IRON DEFICIENCY ANEMIA	BETA-THALASSEMIA MINOR	ANEMIA OF CHRONIC DISEASE
Reticulocyte count	Without reticulocytosis	Without reticulocytosis	Without reticulocytosis
Peripheral smear	Normal or hypochromia and microcytosis	Hypochromia, target cells, microcytes, basophilic stippling	Normal or hypochromia and microcytosis
Serum iron	Low	Normal or high	Low
Iron-binding capacity	High*	Normal	Normal or low
Iron saturation	Low	Normal (20%–55%)	Normal or low
Serum ferritin	Low	Normal or high	Normal or high
RDW	Increased	Normal	Usually normal
Hemoglobin electrophoresis	Normal	Increased HbA$_2$ and HbF	Normal

*>300 μg/dl (54 μmol/L).[1]

IRON DEFICIENCY ANEMIA

Although iron deficiency anemia is typically a microcytic anemia, in mild iron deficiency the erythrocytes may be normocytic. Initially there is a loss of stainable bone marrow iron and a decrease in the serum ferritin level, which is followed by a decrease in serum iron and an increase in the total iron-binding capacity. Then anemia occurs with a decreasing MCV, an increasing poikilocytosis, and hypochromia. The MCV does not usually fall below 80 fl until the hemoglobin falls below 10 g/dl. A decreasing erythrocyte count and an increasing RDW are early changes. In a case of pure iron deficiency, it is unusual to find an erythrocyte count less than 2.5 million. The fall in the erythrocyte count tends to be less than the fall in hemoglobin. Generally, examination of the bone marrow is not required to establish a diagnosis of iron deficiency anemia. An exception is the clinical situation where iron deficiency coexists with a chronic disease.[1,6,11]

The RDW is more accurate than previously used formulas to distinguish iron deficiency anemia from anemia of chronic disease and beta-thalassemia minor. Formulas that have been used to distinguish iron deficiency from beta-thalassemia minor include (1) the Mentzer index (MCV/erythrocyte count), which, if greater than 13, favors iron deficiency anemia and, if less than 13, favors beta-thalassemia minor; and (2) the discriminant function (DF') of England and Fraser (DF' =

MCV $-$ [Hemoglobin $\times$ 5] $-$ Erythrocyte count $-$ 3.4), where a positive number indicates iron deficiency anemia and a negative number indicates beta-thalassemia minor.[11]

BETA-THALASSEMIA MINOR

Beta-thalassemia minor is typically microcytic, and, in contrast to iron deficiency anemia, is characterized by a normal or elevated erythrocyte count; for example, at a hemoglobin level of 9 g/dl, an iron-deficient patient has an erythrocyte count of about 3 million/μl, whereas a patient with beta-thalassemia minor has an erythrocyte count of about 5 million/μl. Although there is variation in cell shape and the cells are small, the variation in size is no more than normal and the RDW is normal. If the hemoglobin level is greater than 10 g/dl but the MCV is less than 75 fl, thalassemia is more likely than iron deficiency anemia. In the case of beta-thalassemia minor, the diagnosis can be established by demonstrating increased levels of hemoglobins A_2 and F using hemoglobin electrophoresis. Sometimes, however, the matter is not so simple, such as with alpha-thalassemia minor (in which hemoglobin electrophoresis is normal), with delta beta-thalassemia, and with concurrent iron deficiency, which are known to prevent the increase in the hemoglobin A_2 level.[1,4,11]

ANEMIA OF CHRONIC DISEASE

The anemia of chronic disease is typically normocytic or mildly microcytic, and the MCV rarely falls below 78 fl. In contrast to iron deficiency anemia, the serum iron is low, iron-binding capacity is normal or low, and the serum ferritin is usually greater than 100 ng/ml. Of course, iron deficiency and anemia of chronic disease may occur together, such as in patients with inflammatory bowel disease, rheumatic diseases treated with aspirin or nonsteroidal anti-inflammatory drugs, or hepatic disease. In these conditions, the iron saturation (iron/total iron-binding capacity) may be quite low, even without iron deficiency. If, however, the saturation is greater than 30%, then iron deficiency is excluded. A serum ferritin level less than 50 ng/ml in these inflammatory conditions suggests iron deficiency. This is because serum ferritin is an acute-phase reactant and tends to be elevated in these chronic inflammatory states. When serum ferritin levels are borderline (50 ng/ml), one may need to obtain a bone marrow aspirate for iron stain to settle the question.[1,6,10,11]

4. In patients with anemia, the following additional abnormal laboratory test results may occur:

CHEMISTRY

- Hypobilirubinemia related to the decreased erythrocyte mass in anemia
- Hypocholesterolemia, possibly related to role of erythrocyte membranes exchanging cholesterol with the plasma

REFERENCES

1. Beutler E: The common anemias. JAMA 259:2433, 1988.
2. Carmel R, Weiner JM, Johnson CS: Iron deficiency occurs frequently in patients with pernicious anemia. JAMA 257:1081, 1987.
3. Finch CA, Bellotti V, Stray S et al: Plasma ferritin determination as a diagnostic tool. West J Med 145:657, 1986.
4. Gehlbach DL, Morgenstern LL: Antenatal screening for thalassemia minor. Obstet Gynecol 71:801, 1988.
5. Griner PF: Iron deficiency anemia. In Griner PF, Panzer RJ, Greenland P: Clinical Diagnosis and the Laboratory: Logical Strategies for Common Medical Problems. Chicago, Year Book Medical Publishers, Inc, 1986, p 431.
6. Hematology Subspecialty Committee: Medical Knowledge Self-Assessment Program VIII. Hematology. Philadelphia, American College of Physicians, 1988, p 461.
7. Psaty BM, Tierney WM, Martin DK, et al: The value of serum iron studies as a test for iron-deficiency anemia in a county hospital. J Gen Intern Med 2:160, 1987.
8. Sears DA: Weakness and joint pains (microcytic anemia without reticulocytosis). In Cutler P: Problem Solving in Clinical Medicine: From Data to Diagnosis, 2nd ed. Baltimore, Williams & Wilkins, 1985, p 227.
9. Simel DL: Is the RDW-MCV classification of anemia useful? Clin Lab Haematol 9:349, 1987.
10. Thompson WG, Meola T, Lipkin M, et al: Red cell distribution width, mean corpuscular volume, and transferrin saturation in the diagnosis of iron deficiency anemia. Arch Intern Med 148:2128, 1988.
11. Wallerstein RO: Laboratory evaluation of anemia. West J Med 146:443, 1987.

INFECTIOUS MONONUCLEOSIS

Infectious mononucleosis (IM) is a clinical syndrome caused by infection with the Epstein-Barr virus (EBV). Other disorders associated with EBV infection include Burkitt's lymphoma, nasopharyngeal carcinoma, and several other lymphoproliferative disorders. IM occurs mainly in individuals 10 to 20 years of age, and approximately 12% of susceptible college-age students seroconvert each year, about 50% of whom develop infectious mononucleosis. Young children usually have mild infections and often do not produce heterophile antibodies, whereas elderly patients may have a persistent febrile syndrome in which the diagnosis is overlooked. Most patients recover in 2 to 3 weeks, although the virus resides in all patients for life. Immunocompromised patients can have overwhelming EBV proliferative syndromes. The disease is passed by oral-oral transmission, rarely by blood transfusion, and probably by sexual contact. Infected B lymphocytes produce a variety of antibodies, including the diagnostic heterophile antibody and antibodies against EBV-associated antigens such as viral capsid antigen (VCA), early antigen (EA), and nuclear antigen (EBNA). Common clinical presentations are pharyngeal (80%), typhoidal (12%), and icteric (8%). Recently, the chronic fatigue syndrome (chronic or recurrent debilitating fatigue plus or minus sore throat, lymphadenitis, headache, myalgia, and arthralgias) has received attention, and a working case definition has been developed.[1-7]

1.   In patients with clinical findings of IM, request a complete blood count (CBC), a leukocyte differential count, and a test for heterophile antibodies.

A CBC and leukocyte differential count are useful to detect the absolute or relative lymphocytosis and atypical lymphocytes that are characteristic of IM. Heterophile antibodies are mixtures of IgG and IgM antibodies that are of a variety of species directed against sheep, horse, and goat erythrocyte membranes. Although stimulated by EBV infection, they are not specific for this infection and can occur after a number of other acute infections. Heterophile antibodies appear 3 days after onset, peak in 2 weeks, remain elevated for 4 to 6 weeks, and then fall and disappear.

2.   Evaluate the tests.

There are a wide variety of heterophile antibody procedures available for IM, most of which are now performed on glass slides or in small tubes. Generally, they differ very little from one another and are quite sensitive and fairly specific in the diagnosis of IM.[6]

3.   If the clinical and hematologic findings are consistent and the heterophile antibody test is positive, conclude that the diagnosis is IM.

The presence of heterophile antibodies in the context of the appropriate clinical and hematologic findings is diagnostic for IM False-positive reactions are rare. Atypical lymphocytes usually account for more than 10% of the leukocytes in the peripheral blood.

4.   If the clinical and hematologic findings are consistent and the heterophile antibody test is negative, consider measuring EBV-specific antibodies. EBV cultures are not usually helpful in making a diagnosis.

Up to 10% of patients with IM are seronegative for heterophile antibodies, and if the clinical course is typical, the presence of heterophile antibodies is not absolutely essential for management. On the other hand, if the patient's course is unusual or puzzling, then measurement of EBV-specific antibodies may be useful. IgM antibodies to VCA indicate acute EBV infection, and IgG antibodies to VCA indicate past infection. Antibodies to EA appear transiently during early infections, and antibodies to EBNA appear late in the course of the illness and persist after recovery. Thus the pattern of EBV-specific antibodies may indicate the stage of the infection. For example, IgM antibodies to VCA and antibodies to EA indicate acute infection, and IgG antibodies to VCA and antibodies to EBNA suggest a past infection.

5.   If heterophile antibodies and EBV-specific antibodies are negative in patients with clinical features of IM, consider other causes for the IM syndrome.

Other infectious agents can cause an IM-like syndrome; the differential diagnosis includes streptococcal or gonococcal pharyngeal infection, cytomegalovirus infection, viral hepatitis, toxoplasmosis, HIV infection, leukemia, and lymphoma.

6. In patients with the chronic fatigue syndrome, measuring EBV-specific antibodies is not usually helpful. Other studies may be appropriate.

Rarely, patients with the chronic fatigue syndrome show a persistently or periodically elevated antibody to EA and a low or absent antibody to EBNA. However, asymptomatic individuals may show similar patterns, and one should be cautious in ascribing the chronic fatigue syndrome to EBV infection. It is likely that, with time, the chronic fatigue syndrome will be shown to have multiple somatic and psychosomatic causes. The Center for Disease Control (CDC)–sponsored case definition requires 2 major and 6 of 14 minor criteria. Major criteria consist of (1) new onset of persisting or relapsing, debilitating fatigue that is not resolved with bed rest and a reduction in daily activity to less than half of the patient's premorbid activity level, for at least 6 months; and (2) exclusion of other known causes of similar symptoms, such as specific infections, neoplasms, psychiatric disorders, or endocrine disease. Minor criteria include mild fever, sore throat, muscle weakness, myalgias, arthralgias, generalized headaches, and neuropsychological symptoms.[4,7]

The role of laboratory tests in the workup of the chronic fatigue syndrome is controversial. Although laboratory tests are not required, the CDC group suggests that, together with the clinical findings, chest radiographs, and intermediate-strength purified protein derivative (PPD) skin test, the following laboratory tests are appropriate: complete blood count (CBC) and differential; erythrocyte sedimentation rate (ESR); serum glucose, urea nitrogen, creatinine, electrolytes, calcium, phosphorus, bilirubin, alkaline phosphatase (ALP), aspartate aminotransferase (AST or SGOT), alanine aminotransferase (ALT or SGPT), creatine phosphokinase (CK) or aldolase, urinalysis, thyroid-stimulating hormone (TSH), antinuclear antibody (ANA), and HIV antibody. Also, serial measurements of weight and morning and afternoon temperatures are indicated.[4]

7. In patients with IM, the following additional abnormal test results may occur:

HEMATOLOGY

- Autoimmune hemolytic anemia caused by cold agglutinins against i antigens
- Leukocyte count may be high, normal, or low; and a relative and absolute neutropenia is present in 60% to 90% of patients
- Thrombocytopenia is common

CHEMISTRY

- Hyperuricemia caused by accelerated lymphocyte nucleic acid turnover
- Increased transaminase levels (AST or SGOT and ALT or SGPT) in about 90% of patients
- Elevated lactate dehydrogenase (LD)
- Increased ALP
- Hyperbilirubinemia, usually mild and only occasionally 6.0 mg/dl (103 μmol/L) or greater; rarely, bilirubin levels of 10.2 to 23.0 mg/dl (174 to 393 μmol/L) may be encountered.[1]

- Depressed serum albumin related to decreased hepatic synthesis
- Elevated serum globulins caused by antibodies to EBV, first IgM and then IgG

REFERENCES

1. Fuhrman SA, Gill R, Howitz CA, et al: Marked hyperbilirubinemia in infectious mononucleosis. Analysis of laboratory data in seven patients. Arch Intern Med 147:850, 1987.
2. Griner PF: Infectious mononucleosis. In Griner PF, Panzer RJ, Greenland P: Clinical Diagnosis and the Laboratory: Logical Strategies for Common Medical Problems. Chicago, Year Book Medical Publishers, Inc, 1986, p 57.
3. Hellinger WC, Smith TF, Van Scoy RE, et al: Chronic fatigue syndrome and the diagnostic utility of antibody to Epstein-Barr virus early antigen. JAMA 260:971, 1988.
4. Holmes GP, Kaplan JE, Gantz NM, et al: Chronic fatigue syndrome: A working case definition. Ann Int Med 108:387, 1988.
5. Kroenke K, Wood DR, Mangelsdorff AD, et al: Chronic fatigue syndrome. Prevalence, patient characteristics, and outcome. JAMA 260:929, 1988.
6. Neff JC: Infectious mononucleosis: A review of the serological diagnosis. University Reference Laboratories Inc, Laboratory Update, January-February, 1988.
7. Swartz MN: The chronic fatigue syndrome—One entity or many? N Engl J Med 319:1728, 1988.

CHAPTER 10

ELECTROLYTE DISORDERS

HYPONATREMIA

Hyponatremia is a hypotonic disorder caused by a depressed serum sodium concentration, below 136 mEq/L (136 mmol/L). The clinical features are produced by brain swelling secondary to a decreased extracellular fluid osmolality. Causes include excessive total body water and sodium depletion. When evaluating hyponatremia, it is important to assess whether the patient is hypervolemic, hypovolemic, or euvolemic. Usually, hyponatremia is modest, the patient is asymptomatic, and if the cause is removed (e.g., diuretic therapy), the condition improves. On the other hand, severe symptomatic hyponatremia (serum sodium <120 mEq/L [120 mmol/L]) is rare but constitutes a medical emergency. The findings progress from lethargy, weakness, and somnolence to seizures, coma, and death as the hyponatremia worsens.[1-8]

1.   In patients with hyponatremia or clinical findings of hyponatremia, rule out pseudohyponatremia before proceeding with the workup. Request measurements of serum sodium and osmolality and urine sodium.

A serum sodium determination can verify the hyponatremia, and serum osmolality and urine sodium measurments are useful to determine the cause of the hyponatremia. Drugs may be a contributing factor.

Serum or heparinized plasma is satisfactory, but avoid sodium salts of heparin. When obtaining the blood specimen, avoid significant hemolysis, which can decrease the serum sodium concentration because of a dilutional effect from the erythrocyte fluid. Lipemia or hyperproteinemia can artifactually decrease the serum sodium level, causing a normal serum sodium level to appear decreased.

2.   Evaluate the tests.

Rule out pseudohyponatremia (euosmolar hyponatremia) caused by severe hyperlipidemia or hyperproteinemia. If the serum is lipemic or the proteins are high,* determine whether there is a significant osmolal gap according to the following formula:

Osmolal gap = Measured osmolality − Calculated osmolality (all units in mOsm/kg)

where:

$$\text{Calculated osmolality (mOsm/kg)} = 2 \times \text{Na (mEq/L)} + \frac{\text{Glucose (mg/dl)}}{18} + \frac{\text{Urea (mg/dl)}}{2.8}$$

---

*Proteins usually greater than 10 g/dl, a concentration encountered almost exclusively in patients with multiple myeloma.

149

or

Calculated osmolality (mOsm/kg) = 2 × Na (mmol/L) +
Glucose (mmol/L) + Urea nitrogen (mmol/L)

TEST	SPECIMEN	REFERENCE RANGE (CONVENTIONAL)	REFERENCE RANGE (INTERNATIONAL)
Osmolality	Serum	275–295 mOsm/kg of water	275–295 mOsm/kg of water

The occurrence of pseudohyponatremia is method dependent; that is, it is observed when the serum sodium is measured by flame photometry but not when it is measured in undiluted serum by an ion-specific electrode. It is important to recognize pseudohyponatremia, since, because serum osmolality is normal, no therapy is required.

If the measured osmolality is normal and there is a significant osmolal gap, the low serum sodium is probably an artifact caused by lipemia or hyperproteinemia. This is true only if there is no unusual osmotically active substance (ethanol, methanol, mannitol) in the serum, because these substances can also cause an increased osmolal gap (see the discussion of alcoholism in Chapter 2).

A high serum glucose (an osmotically active, low-molecular solute) can also contribute to a low serum sodium, and every 100 mg/dl (5.55 mmol/L) rise in the serum glucose produces a decline of approximately 1.6 mEq/L (1.6 mmol/L) in the serum sodium level.[7] This phenomenon can also occur with mannitol. Increased serum immunoglobulins, particularly IgG (but also IgA), can behave as cations and cause a decreased serum sodium level and a low anion gap [Anion gap = Na − (Cl + HCO_3)]. Normally, the gap is 8 to 14 mEq/L (8 to 14 mmol/L) and is composed of phosphate, sulfate, organic acids, and proteinate. Myeloma patients have a mean anion gap of 6.8, whereas the mean gap of controls is 9.4; patients with monoclonal gammopathy of undetermined significance have a mean anion gap of 9.1.[5]

In true hyponatremia the severity of the clinical findings correlates with the degree of hyponatremia and the rate at which it develops. In acute hyponatremia, the clinical features generally appear when the serum sodium concentration falls to 120 mEq/L (120 mmol/L) or less. In chronic hyponatremia, clinical manifestations are far less common, even when the serum sodium concentration is below 120 mEq/L (120 mmol/L).

Be careful not to correct severe hyponatremia too aggressively, since this has been reported to cause central pontine myelinolysis.[1]

3. Interpret test results in the context of clinical findings.

WATER INTAKE AND DRUGS

Certain drugs, such as diuretics and agents that induce the syndrome of inappropriate secretion of antidiuretic hormone (SIADH), can cause a decreased serum sodium level. There is a syndrome of thiazide-induced SIADH in which hyponatremia, hypokalemia, and metabolic alkalosis occur together. Drugs that can induce SIADH include oral hypoglycemic agents, antineoplastic and immunosuppressive agents, psychoactive drugs, and clofibrate. Excessive water intake, such as in psychogenic polydipsia, can cause hyponatremia.

DILUTIONAL HYPONATREMIA

Dilutional hyponatremia in which there is an excess of total body sodium and water with edema and ascites occurs in congestive heart failure, cirrhosis, and the nephrotic syndrome. Increased water intake, marked sodium restriction, or diuretic therapy, or all three may aggravate any of these conditions.

HYPONATREMIA FROM SODIUM DEPLETION

In hyponatremia from sodium depletion, there is neither edema nor ascites. Clinical features of extracellular volume depletion are present. These include tachycardia, decreased central venous pressure, an elevated hematocrit, and elevated serum proteins. If the urine sodium concentration is below 10 mEq/L (10 mmol/L) (the serum chloride is usually low), possible causes include gastrointestinal losses, excessive perspiration with replacement of water but not enough sodium, and volume depletion without replacement of water and electrolytes after diuretic therapy. If the urine sodium is above 10 mEq/L (10 mmol/L), causes include adrenocortical insufficiency and salt-losing nephropathy.

OTHER CAUSES OF HYPONATREMIA

Other causes of hyponatremia that are not associated with edema or volume depletion include the SIADH (from malignant tumors, such as carcinoma of the lung or pancreas; central nervous system disorders, such as tumors, infections, hemorrhages, and cerebrovascular thrombosis; and pulmonary disorders, such as tuberculosis, abscess, and viral, bacterial, or fungal pneumonia), hypothyroidism, and essential hyponatremia, which often occurs in the context of chronic illness.

REFERENCES

1. Ashouri OS: Severe diuretic-induced hyponatremia in the elderly. A series of eight patients. Arch Intern Med 146:1355, 1986.
2. Ayus JC: Diuretic-induced hyponatremia. Arch Intern Med 146:1295, 1986.
3. Contiguglia SR, Mishell JL, Klein MH: Hyponatremia. In Friedman H (ed): Problem-Oriented Medical Diagnosis, 3rd ed. Boston, Little, Brown & Co, 1983, p 251.
4. Cutler P: Weakness and disorientation (hyponatremia). In Cutler P: Problem Solving in Clinical Medicine: From Data to Diagnosis, 2nd ed. Baltimore, Williams & Wilkins, 1985, p 459.
5. Flanagan NG, Ridway JC, Irving AG: The anion gap as a screening procedure for occult myeloma in the elderly. J Roy Soc Med 81:27, 1988.
6. Kassirer JP, Hricik DE, Cohen JJ: Repairing Body Fluids. Principles and Practice. Philadelphia, WB Saunders Co, 1989, p 27.

7. Moran SM, Jamison RL: The variable hyponatremic response to hyperglycemia. West J Med 142:49, 1985.
8. Walmsley RN, White GH: Hyponatremia. In Pocket Diagnostic Clinical Chemistry. Melbourne, Blackwell Scientific Publication, 1985, p 15.

HYPERNATREMIA

Hypernatremia is a hypertonic disorder caused by an elevated serum sodium concentration, above 146 mEq/L (146 mmol/L). The clinical features are produced by brain shrinkage secondary to an increased extracellular fluid osmolality. Causes include too much dietary salt, too little dietary water, or excessive water loss from the body. Clinical findings of hypernatremia progress from somnolence, confusion, and coma to respiratory paralysis and death as the hypernatremia worsens.[1-6]

1. In patients with hypernatremia or clinical findings of hypernatremia, request measurements of serum sodium and serum and urine osmolality.

A serum sodium determination can verify the hypernatremia, and serum and urine osmolality measurements are helpful to determine the cause of the hypernatremia. Dietary sodium, water, and drugs may be contributing factors.

The specimen collection and handling considerations are the same as for hyponatremia.

2. Evaluate the tests.

The severity of the clinical findings correlates with the degree of hypernatremia and the rate at which it develops. In acute hypernatremia, symptoms may appear when serum osmolality exceeds 320 to 330 mOsm/kg, and respiratory arrest may appear when it exceeds 360 to 380 mOsm/kg.

In diabetics, nonketotic hyperglycemic hyperosmolality can produce clinical findings similar to hypernatremia. In this syndrome, the serum sodium is initially low, but as hyperglycemia rapidly depletes extracellular water, the serum sodium may become normal or elevated. Depressed consciousness is uncommon when serum osmolality is less than 350 mOsm/kg, whereas virtually all patients with serum osmolalities exceeding 400 mOsm/kg are comatose.[4]

3. Interpret test results in the context of clinical findings.

WATER INTAKE AND DRUGS

Certain drugs, such as mineralocorticoids or osmotic diuretics, can cause an increased serum sodium level. Other causes include excessive salt intake relative to water intake, which is unusual. Examples include inadvertent feeding of infants with high-sodium content foods and hyperalimentation of patients by intravenous or nasogastric tube feeding with preparations containing too much sodium. Inadequate water intake may occur with impaired thirst, such as occurs in mentally obtunded patients.

EXCESSIVE WATER LOSS

If the urine is hyperosmotic (maximally concentrated), consider excessive water loss caused by gastrointestinal disorders (vomiting and diarrhea), hyperpnea, excessive sweating (fever), and burns. If the urine is isosmotic or hyposmotic, consider excessive water loss from chronic renal failure, diuresis after relief of urinary tract obstruction, diuretic phase of acute tubular necrosis, hypercalcemic nephropathy, hypokalemic nephropathy, osmotic diuresis of diabetes mellitus or secondary to urea, and diabetes insipidus (central after cerebral trauma or neurosurgical procedures; and nephrogenic). Hypernatremia caused by a urea diuresis may develop when patients who are unable to complain of thirst are placed on a high-protein feeding.

OTHER CAUSES OF HYPERNATREMIA

In patients with adrenal hyperfunction, mineralocorticoid excess can cause hypernatremia. Hypernatremia above 150 mEq/L (150 mmol/L) can be induced by maximal exercise; the mechanism is unknown.[3] There is also an entity called essential hypernatremia, in which a slightly elevated serum sodium level occurs in the conscious state in a relatively healthy individual. Rule out CNS tumors, CNS granulomas, and cerebrovascular accidents before making a diagnosis of essential hypernatremia. Iatrogenic hypernatremia may occur in elderly patients and is often a marker of severe associated systemic illness.[1,4,5]

REFERENCES

1.   Beck LH: Geriatric hypernatremia. Ann Int Med 107:768, 1987.
2.   Contiguglia SR, Mishell JL, Klein MH: Hypernatremia. In Friedman H (ed): Problem-Oriented Medical Diagnosis, 3rd ed. Boston, Little, Brown & Co, 1983, p 250.
3.   Felig P, Johnson C, Levitt M, et al: Hypernatremia induced by maximal exercise. JAMA 248:1209, 1982.
4.   Kassirer JP, Hricik DE, Cohen JJ: Repairing Body Fluids. Principles and Practice. Philadelphia, WB Saunders, 1989, p 38.
5.   Snyder NA, Feigal DW, Arieff AI: Hypernatremia in elderly patients. A heterogeneous, morbid, and iatrogenic entity. Ann Int Med 107:309, 1987.
6.   Walmsley RN, White GH: Hypernatremia. In Pocket Diagnostic Clinical Chemistry. Melbourne, Blackwell Scientific Publications, 1985, p 13.

HYPOKALEMIA

Hypokalemia is a depressed serum potassium concentration, below 3.5 mEq/L (3.5 mmol/L). The normal serum potassium concentration is greater than the plasma concentration because of the release of platelet potassium during clotting. The most significant effects of hypokalemia relate to neuromuscular and electrocardiographic disturbances. The causes of hypokalemia include diuretic therapy, inadequate potassium intake, excessive renal loss, excessive gastrointestinal loss, and shifts from the extracellular fluid to the intracellular fluid. Clinical features include skeletal muscle weakness and paralysis and derangements in cardiac conduction.[1-5]

1. In patients with hypokalemia or clinical findings of hypokalemia, request a measurement of serum potassium. Consider measuring the 24-hour urinary excretion of potassium to document potassium depletion of renal origin.

A serum potassium determination can verify the hypokalemia, and measurement of urinary potassium excretion can be useful to determine the cause of hypokalemia.

The specimen collection and handling considerations are the same as for hyperkalemia.

2. Evaluate the tests.

At serum potassium concentrations of 2 to 2.5 mEq/L (2 to 2.5 mmol/L), muscular weakness can occur. At lower levels, areflexic paralysis can occur with associated respiratory insufficiency and death. Electrocardiographic manifestations of hypokalemia include sagging of the ST segment, depression of the T wave, and elevation of the U wave. With marked hypokalemia, the T wave becomes progressively smaller and the U wave shows increasing amplitude. In patients treated with digitalis, hypokalemia may precipitate serious arrhythmias.

3. Interpret test results in the context of clinical findings.

Certain drugs, such as the thiazides or loop diuretics, can cause a decreased serum potassium level. Other causes of hypokalemia include **inadequate intake and excessive renal loss,** such as in mineralocorticoid excess (primary or exogenous, and licorice ingestion), Bartter's syndrome, osmotic diuresis, chronic metabolic alkalosis, with certain antibiotics (penicillin-like antibiotics, amphotericin B, gentamicin), renal tubular acidosis, leukemia, Liddle's syndrome, and magnesium depletion; **excessive gastrointestinal loss,** such as vomiting, diarrhea, secretory diarrhea, chronic laxative abuse, villous adenoma, fistulas, ureterosigmoidostomy, and inflammatory bowel disease; and **shifts from the extracellular fluid to the intracellular fluid,** such as in hypokalemic periodic paralysis, ingestion of barium salts, insulin therapy, vitamin B_{12} therapy, epinephrine administration, and metabolic alkalosis.

REFERENCES

1. Contiguglia SR, Mishell JL, Klein MH: Hypokalemia. In Friedman H (ed): Problem-Oriented Medical Diagnosis, 3rd ed. Boston, Little, Brown & Co, 1983, p 253.
2. Cutler P: Fatigue and abnormal ECG (hypokalemia). In Cutler P: Problem Solving in Clinical Medicine: From Data to Diagnosis, 2nd ed. Baltimore, Williams & Wilkins, 1985, p 449.
3. Kassirer JP, Hricik DE, Cohen JJ: Repairing Body Fluids. Principles and Practice. Philadelphia, WB Saunders, 1989, p 46.

4. Stein J: Hypokalemia. Common and uncommon causes. Hosp Pract 23:55, 1988.
5. Walmsley RN, White GH: Hypokalemia. In Pocket Diagnostic Clinical Chemistry. Melbourne, Blackwell Scientific Publications, 1985, p 23.

HYPERKALEMIA

Hyperkalemia is an increased serum potassium concentration, above 5.1 mEq/L (5.1 mmol/L). Normally, the serum potassium concentration is higher than the plasma concentration because of release of platelet potassium during clotting. The most important clinical features of hyperkalemia relate to alterations of cardiac excitability as manifested in the electrocardiogram and depression of neuromuscular activity. Causes of hyperkalemia include excessive intake of potassium, decreased excretion, and shifts of potassium from cells to extracellular fluid. Clinical features include cardiotoxic effects and depressive effects on skeletal muscle.[1-4]

1. In patients with hyperkalemia or clinical findings of hyperkalemia, request a measurement of serum potassium. Rule out artifactual hyperkalemia before proceeding with the workup.

A serum potassium determination can verify the hyperkalemia. Artifactually high serum potassium levels can result from thrombocytosis, leukocytosis, hemolysis, and allowing the serum to remain in contact with the clot for prolonged periods of time at room temperature. Serum or heparinized plasma can be used for potassium measurements, but avoid potassium salts of heparin and promptly separate the serum/plasma from the cells. Opening and closing the fist before venipuncture should be avoided, since the muscle action can result in increased potassium levels of 10% to 20%.

2. Evaluate the tests.

The earliest electrocardiographic manifestation of hyperkalemia consists of peaked T waves and occurs when the serum level exceeds 6.5 mEq/L (6.5 mmol/L). Between 7 and 8 mEq/L (7 and 8 mmol/L) the PR interval is prolonged followed by a loss of P waves and widening of the QRS complex. When the serum potassium level exceeds 8 to 10 mEq/L (8 to 10 mmol/L), a sine wave pattern can develop and cardiac asystole or ventricular fibrillation can occur. Rarely, skeletal muscle weakness and flaccid paralysis can occur. Hyponatremia and acidosis can potentiate the adverse effects of hyperkalemia on the heart.

3. Interpret test results in the context of clinical findings.

Certain drugs, such as antineoplastic agents, heparin, and potassium-sparing diuretics (triamterene, spironolactone), can cause an increased serum potassium level. Other causes of hyperkalemia include **excessive intake,** especially in renal insufficiency; **increased cellular release of potassium,** such as in metabolic acidosis, trauma, burns, rhabdomyolysis, hemolysis, tumorlysis, drugs (succinylcholine, digitalis, beta-blocking agents), hyperosmolality, insulin deficiency, hyperkalemic periodic paralysis, and severe muscle disease; and **decreased renal excretion of potassium,** such as in acute oliguric renal failure, chronic renal failure, renal tubular disorders, Addison's disease, and hypoaldosteronism.

REFERENCES

1. Alvo M, Warnock DG: Hyperkalemia (Medical Staff Conference). West J Med 141:666, 1984.
2. Contiguglia SR, Mishell JL, Klein MH: Hyperkalemia. In Friedman H (ed): Problem-Oriented Medical Diagnosis, 3rd ed. Boston, Little, Brown & Co, 1983, p 252.
3. Kassirer JP, Hricik DE, Cohen JJ: Repairing Body Fluids. Principles and Practice. Philadelphia, WB Saunders, 1989, p 60.
4. Walmsley RN, White GH: Hyperkalemia. In Pocket Diagnostic Clinical Chemistry. Melbourne, Blackwell Scientific Publications, 1985, p 25.

HYPOPHOSPHATEMIA

Hypophosphatemia is a decreased serum phosphate concentration, below 2.7 mg/dl (0.87 mmol/L). The clinical features are produced by a deficiency of phosphorus for key metabolic functions, including the integrity of all cell membranes, the structure of nucleic acids, a second messenger in endocrinology (cAMP, cGMP), the release of oxygen by hemoglobin (2,3-DPG), and the buffering of urine. Causes include decreased intake of phosphate, impaired absorption of phosphate, excessive renal loss of phosphate, and a shift of phosphate into cells and bone. The diagnosis of hypophosphatemia and its cause depends on obtaining appropriate tests in the context of the clinical findings. These findings include red cell dysfunction and hemolysis, leukocyte dysfunction, platelet dysfunction, weakness, congestive cardiomyopathy, rhabdomyolysis, central nervous system dysfunction, and possible hepatic dysfunction.[1-7]

1. In patients with hypophosphatemia or clinical findings of hypophosphatemia, request a serum phosphorous measurement. Consider obtaining a complete blood count (CBC), serum glucose, urea nitrogen, creatinine, calcium, creatine kinase, liver function tests, and urinalysis.

A serum phosphorous determination can verify the hypophosphatemia. A CBC can detect hemolytic anemia and thrombocytopenia. Serum glucose can assess carbohydrate homeostasis; and serum urea nitrogen, creatinine, and a urinalysis can determine renal function. The serum creatine kinase can detect cardiac or skeletal muscle damage, and liver function tests can assess hepatic function.

Serum or heparinized plasma is satisfactory. The patient should be fasting, since postprandial phosphorylation of glucose decreases serum phosphorus.

Collection of the specimen after an overnight fast is ideal. Hemolysis and prolonged contact with the clot should be avoided, because it will increase serum phosphorus.

2. Evaluate the tests.

It is unusual for hypophosphatemia to cause metabolic disturbances at concentrations above 1.5 mg/dl (0.48 mmol/L). If concentrations are below 1.5 mg/dl and you decide to treat with parenteral phosphate, be careful, since hyperphosphatemia can result and ionized calcium can fall, producing tetany or convulsions. In addition, metastatic calcifications of soft tissues can occur.

3. Interpret test results in the context of clinical findings.

Certain drugs, such as steroids, diuretics, and insulin, can decrease serum phosphorus. Vomiting and prolonged nasogastric suction can limit phosphorous intake. Other causes include **decreased phosphate intake; impaired phosphate absorption** with drugs (aluminum- and magnesium-containing antacids) and in alcoholism; **excessive renal loss of phosphate,** as in hyperparathyroidism, renal tubular disorders, and acidosis; and **intracellular shifts of phosphate,** as in carbohydrate loading, hyperalimentation, respiratory alkalosis, rapid tumor growth, the nutritional recovery syndrome, burns, and the hungry bone syndrome (hypocalcemia and hypophosphatemia caused by bone remineralization after parathyroid surgery).[1]

REFERENCES

1. Brasier AR, Nussbaum SR: Hungry bone syndrome: Clinical and biochemical predictors of its occurrence after parathyroid surgery. Am J Med 84:654, 1988.
2. Contiguglia SR, Mishell JL, Klein MH: Hypophosphatemia. In Friedman H (ed): Problem-Oriented Medical Diagnosis, 3rd ed. Boston, Little, Brown & Co, 1983, p 254.
3. Kassirer JP, Hricik DE, Cohen JJ: Repairing Body Fluids. Principles and Practice. Philadelphia, WB Saunders, 1989, p 109.
4. Knochel JP: The clinical status of hypophosphatemia. An update. N Engl J Med 313:447, 1985.
5. Morris RC: Moderate hypophosphatemia—Not always an innocent bystander. West J Med 147:577, 1987.
6. Walmsley RN, White GH: Hypophosphatemia. In Pocket Diagnostic Clinical Chemistry. Melbourne, Blackwell Scientific Publications, 1985, p 73.
7. Yu GC, Lee DBN: Clinical disorders of phosphorous metabolism. West J Med 147:569, 1987.

HYPERPHOSPHATEMIA

Hyperphosphatemia is an elevated serum phosphate concentration, above 4.5 mg/dl (1.45 mmol/L). When severe, hyperphosphatemia can contribute to the acidosis of uremia, further reduce the concentration of ionized calcium in the extracellular fluid, and cause metastatic calcification in soft tissues. The most common cause is renal insufficiency. Hyperphosphatemia produces no direct clinical symptoms.[1-4]

1. In patients with hyperphosphatemia, request a determination of serum phosphorus. Consider obtaining measurements of serum calcium, glucose, urea nitrogen, and creatinine and a urinalysis.

A serum phosphorous determination can verify the hyperphosphatemia. Hypocalcemia may be a clue to hypoparathyroidism; hyperglycemia a clue to acromegaly; and urea nitrogen, creatinine, and urinalysis an indication of renal insufficiency.

Specimen collection and handling are the same as for hypophosphatemia.

2. Evaluate the tests.

Hyperphosphatemia can indirectly produce tetany by lowering serum calcium. With rapid elevations of serum phosphorus, hypocalcemia and tetany may occur with a serum phosphorous concentration as low as 6 mg/dl (1.94 mmol/L), a level that, if reached more slowly, has no detectable effect on serum calcium.[2]

3. Interpret test results in the context of clinical findings.

Certain drugs, such as steroids and thiazides, can increase the serum phosphate level. If truly large amounts of phosphate are administered orally, parenterally, or rectally, hyperphosphatemia can occur even in the presence of normal renal function. **Other causes of hyperphosphatemia** include increased tubular reabsorption (hypoparathyroidism, pseudohypoparathyroidism, acromegaly, hyperthyroidism, tumoral calcinosis), transcellular shifts (acidosis), cell lysis (rhabdomyolysis, hemolysis, chemotherapy, malignant pyrexia), and miscellaneous factors (e.g., familial intermittent hyperphosphatemia).

REFERENCES

1. Contiguglia SR, Mishell JL, Klein MH: Hyperphosphatemia. In Friedman H (ed): Problem-Oriented Medical Diagnosis, 3rd ed. Boston, Little, Brown & Co, 1983, p 254.
2. Kassirer JP, Hricik DE, Cohen JJ: Repairing Body Fluids. Principles and Practice. Philadelphia, WB Saunders, 1989, p 102.
3. Walmsley RN, White GH: Hyperphosphatemia. In Pocket Diagnostic Clinical Chemistry. Melbourne, Blackwell Scientific Publications, 1985, p 71.
4. Yu GC, Lee DBN: Clinical disorders of phosphorous metabolism. West J Med 147:569, 1987.

HYPOMAGNESEMIA

Hypomagnesemia is a depression of the serum magnesium concentration to below 1.3 mEq/L (0.65 mmol/L). It is more common than hypermagnesemia and usually occurs as a component of a more complex deficiency state. Low levels of magnesium ions cause hyperirritability of nerves and muscles with manifestations in the neuromuscular, cardiovascular, and gastrointestinal systems. Causes of hypomagnesemia include decreased absorption from dietary sources, increased loss from the body, and internal redistributions. Clinical manifestations include lethargy, weakness, irritability, short attention span, fainting, convulsions, and Chvostek's and Trousseau's signs. There may be anorexia, nausea, vomiting, paralytic ileus, and cardiac arrhythmias.[1-7]

1. In patients with hypomagnesemia or clinical findings of hypomagnesemia, request measurements of serum magnesium, calcium, and potassium.

A serum magnesium determination can verify the hypomagnesemia. Measurements of calcium and potassium can be helpful, because hypocalcemia and hypokalemia frequently accompany hypomagnesemia. The hypocalcemia and hypokalemia may be resistant to treatment unless the hypomagnesemia is corrected first. Routine determinations of serum magnesium are unnecessary in patients with uncomplicated hypertension who are receiving triamterene-containing diuretics or low-dose (50 mg/day or less) hydrochlorothiazide.[4]

2. Evaluate the tests.

Clinical findings increase in number and severity as the serum magnesium becomes progressively decreased. Values of 1.2 mEq/L (0.60 mmol/L) or lower are associated with weakness, irritability, tetany, and convulsions.

3. Interpret test results in the context of clinical findings.

Certain drugs, such as diuretics, can decrease the serum magnesium level. Other causes include **decreased absorption from dietary sources,** as in a low magnesium diet, inhibition of absorption by ethanol, malabsorption, uremia, and selective defect in magnesium absorption (rare); **increased magnesium loss,** as in gastrointestinal disorders (diarrhea) and renal disorders (tubular defects); and **internal redistribution of magnesium,** as in acute pancreatitis and increased loss into bone.

REFERENCES

1. Contiguglia SR, Mishell JL, Klein MH: Hypomagnesemia. In Friedman H (ed): Problem-Oriented Medical Diagnosis, 3rd ed. Boston, Little, Brown & Co, 1983, p 255.
2. Elin RJ: Assessment of magnesium status. Clin Chem 33:1965, 1987.
3. Kassirer JP, Hricik DE, Cohen JJ: Repairing Body Fluids. Principles and Practice. Philadelphia, WB Saunders, 1989, p 118.
4. Kroenke K, Wood DR, Hanley JF: The value of serum magnesium determinations in hypertensive patients receiving diuretics. Arch Intern Med 147:1553, 1987.
5. Reinhart RA: Magnesium metabolism. A review with special reference to the relationship between intracellular content and serum levels. Arch Intern Med 148:2415, 1988.
6. Speicher CE: Magnesium. Clinical Chemistry No. CC-119. Chicago, American Society of Clinical Pathologists, 1979.
7. Walmsley RN, White GH: Hypomagnesemia. In Pocket Diagnostic Clinical Chemistry. Melbourne, Blackwell Scientific Publications, 1985, p 75.

HYPERMAGNESEMIA

Hypermagnesemia is an elevation of the serum magnesium concentration above 2.1 mEq/L (1.05 mmol/L). The magnesium ion exerts a depressive effect on the neuromuscular junction, and the clinical manifestations of hypermagnesemia are related to toxic effects on the central nervous and cardiovascular systems. Hypermagnesemia occurs in patients with renal insufficiency who ingest excessive amounts of magnesium, such as in magnesium-containing antacids. It can result from parenteral administration of magnesium, such as in the treatment of acute hypertension. Clinical manifestations include hypotension and cardiac arrhythmias. The cardiotoxicity of magnesium is aggravated by hypocalcemia, hyperkalemia, acidosis, digitalis therapy, and renal insufficiency (beyond its effect on the magnesium level).[1-6,X]

1. In patients with hypermagnesemia or clinical findings of hypermagnesemia, measure serum magnesium, urea nitrogen, creatinine, calcium, and potassium.

A serum magnesium determination can verify the hypermagnesemia. Measurements of calcium and potassium can be helpful because of the synergistic effects of hypocalcemia and hyperkalemia. Serum urea nitrogen and creatinine are useful to assess renal function.

2. Evaluate the tests.

The cardiac effects of magnesium usually begin at levels greater than 10 mEq/L (5 mmol/L) and consist of peripheral vasodilation with hypotension, depression of the cardiac conduction system, bradyrhythmias, and cardiac arrest in asystole, with more serious effects at higher levels, such as asystole at levels above 25 mEq/L (12.50 mmol/L). Occasionally, patients develop cardiotoxicity at 4.5 to 5.5 mEq/L (2.25 to 2.75 mmol/L).

3. Interpret test results in the context of clinical findings.

Certain drugs, such as magnesium-containing medications, can increase the serum magnesium level. **Another common cause of hypermagnesemia** is renal insufficiency. Miscellaneous causes of mild hypermagnesemia include Addison's disease, diabetic ketoacidosis, hypothyroidism, pituitary dwarfism, lithium therapy, viral hepatitis, and the milk-alkali syndrome.[3]

REFERENCES

1. Contiguglia SR, Mishell JL, Klein MH: Hypermagnesemia. In Friedman H (ed): Problem-Oriented Medical Diagnosis, 3rd ed. Boston, Little, Brown & Co, 1983, p 255.
2. Elin RJ: Assessment of magnesium status. Clin Chem 33:1965, 1987.
3. Kassirer JP, Hricik DE, Cohen JJ: Repairing Body Fluids. Principles and Practice. Philadelphia, WB Saunders, 1989, p 126.
4. Reinhart RA: Magnesium metabolism. A review with special reference to the relationship between intracellular content and serum levels. Arch Intern Med 148:2415, 1988.

5. Speicher CE: Magnesium. Clinical Chemistry No. CC-119. Chicago, American Society of Clinical Pathologists, 1979.
6. Walmsley RN, White GH: Hypermagnesemia. In Pocket Diagnostic Clinical Chemistry. Melbourne, Blackwell Scientific Publications, 1985, p 76.

GENERAL REFERENCE

I. Branch WT (ed): Office Practice of Medicine, 2nd ed. Philadelphia, W Saunders, 1987.

II. Braunwald E, Isselbacher KJ, Petersdorf RG, et al (eds): Harrison's Principles of Internal Medicine, 11th ed. New York, McGraw-Hill Book Co, 1987.

III. Friedman RB, Anderson RE, Entine SM, et al: Effects of diseases on clinical laboratory tests. Clin Chem 26:1D, 1980.

IV. Henry JB (ed): Clinical Diagnosis and Management by Laboratory Methods, 17th ed. Philadelphia, WB Saunders, 1984.

V. Rubenstein E, Federman DD (eds): Scientific American Medicine. New York, Scientific American, 1988.

VI. Speicher CE, Smith JW: Choosing Effective Laboratory Tests. Philadelphia, WB Saunders, 1983.

VII. Statland BE: Clinical Decision Levels for Lab Tests. Oradell, NJ, Medical Economics Books, 1983.

VIII. Wallach J: Interpretation of Diagnostic Tests. A Synopsis of Laboratory Medicine, 4th ed. Boston, Little, Brown & Co, 1986.

IX. Wolf PL: Intepretation of Biochemical Multitest Profiles. An Analysis of 100 Important Conditions. New York, Masson Publishing USA, Inc, 1977.

X. Wyngaarden JB, Smith LH (eds): Cecil Textbook of Medicine, 18th ed. Philadelphia, WB Saunders, 1988.

INDEX